The Mirror of Stones

THE
MIRROR
OF
STONES:

IN WHICH

The Nature, Generation, Properties, Virtues and various Species of more than 200 different Jewels, precious and rare Stones, are distinctly described.

Also certain and infallible Rules to know the Good from the Bad, how to prove their Genuineness, and to distinguish the Real from Counterfeits.

Extracted from the Works of *Aristotle, Pliny, Isiodorus, Dionysius Alexandrinus, Albertus Magnus,* &c.

By *Camillus Leonardus*, M. D.

A Treatise of infinite Use, not only to Jewellers, Lapidaries, and Merchants who trade in them, but to the Nobility and Gentry, who purchase them either for Curiosity, Use, or Ornament.

Dedicated by the Author to C Æ S A R B O R G I A

Now first Translated into *English*.

L O N D O N
Printed for *J. Freeman* in *Fleet street*, 1750

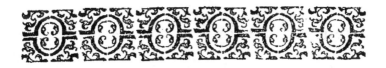

Camillus Leonardus,

Phyſician, of *Piſaro,*

TO THE

Moſt Illuſtrious and moſt Glorious Prince,

Cæſar Borgia,

Of *France,* Duke of *Romandiola,*

Wiſhes Health and Proſperity.

ALtho' we are well aſſured that your Highneſs, in this tempeſtuous Seaſon, is burden'd with the many and weighty Affairs of the Wars: Yet as you are wont, from your innate Goodneſs, Prudence, and Love of Letters and honeſt Arts, with which you are ſo eminently adorned, not only readily to hear, but heartily embrace learned Men, and thoſe who apply themſelves

to

to virtuous Purfuits, we made no Scruple
to fend you this little Book, with this
View, that you may refrefh your Mind,
wearied with perpetual Sollicitudes and
Labours, with the Novelty of a Work,
which, we prefume, will not be wholly
unprofitable, and will yield fome Pleafure
in the Perufal. But how little we are at
Leifure, moft renowned Prince, your
whole City of *Pifaro* can teftify: For being devoted to the Practice of Phyfick and
Speculation, we very willingly apply our
whole Care, Thoughts, Studies and Labours, Day and Night, to the Health of its
Citizens. Being therefore thus encumber'd
with thefe and other Employments both
publick and private, you may eafily judge
how feldom we are at Liberty. Never-
thelefs, if, in the mean Time, any Cef-
fation from Bufinefs happens, we very
chearfully employ fuch an Interval in Li-
terary Studies, and as we are obliged by
the common Ties of our Office, fo it
has been our conftant Practice, according
to our Ability, to promote the Benefit
and Utility of Mankind. Being govern'd
by thefe Motives, we have compofed this
little Treatife of the Nature of fuch Stones

as contribute to the Health or Usefulness
of Men, tho' at the Expence of late
Hours, much Labour, and diligent Enquiries, and tho' the Materials of it were
dispersed thro' the Volumes of various
Authors. We have, however, with the
utmost Care, Labour and Attention, collected such Things as have been handled
in the Writings of the most famous Men,
into this small Tract, which we have en-
titled The Mirror of Stones: In
which, as in a Looking-glass, we may
behold their Nature, Powers and Sculptures, and attain to the Knowledge of
many Things. But we, who are bound
both by Faith and Duty to your High-
ness, in whom our Hope is placed, who
art as well the Father as the Prince of
your Country, to your Name we have
inscribed this Book, and this the rather,
as you are studious, and not only devote
yourself with all your Might to Arms
and the Military, but also to the Liberal
Arts. Now if you should happen, at a
vacant Hour, to cast your Eye over it,
and should find any Thing injudiciously
express'd, and not approved by your dif-
cerning Judgment, be pleased to ascribe

it

it to the Poorness of our Wit, and grant us your Pardon ; for we are not all alike capable of all Things; but where you shall find any Thing worth your Reading, that you will attribute it to those most worthy Doctors from whose Writings we have extracted it , in Regard to whose high Authority and respectable Dignity, you will not disdain to give our little Book a Place, and number it among the, I had almost said, innumerable Volumes of your most excellent Library, that when you look upon it. your Love for CAMILLUS, the Author of it, may be the more ardent. Small, indeed, most glorious and magnanimous Prince, will this Present be in Return for those invaluable Favours you have confer'd upon us But, according to your usual Clemency and Benignity, you will consider, not so much this Trifle of a Book, and the Contents of its Sheets, as the Mind and Good-will of the Author Farewel, and may you long be happy.

Pisaro, the Ides of *September*, in the Year of Salvation, MCCCCCII

The **Translator's**

PREFACE.

*I*F *the Value of a Book was to be rated by the Scarcity of it, I am apt to think, that there is not a Librarian in* Europe *can shew one, of equal Bulk, that has a better Title to the Choice of the Curious, than this* MIRROR OF STONES. *For tho' the Number of its Pages are but* 244, *in a small* Octavo, *and printed in a large Letter, yet there is wrote on the Cover of that which by a peculiar Favour I am possessed of,* This is a scarce Book, and has been valued at 100 Piftoles. *A certain Nobleman, who is pleas'd to honour me with his Friendship,*

A 4 *sought*

fought for it in vain in the moſt noted Libraries in England, *but being determined to have it if there was one in* Europe, *ſent a Gentleman to* France, *where he was to make the leſt Enquiry he was able among the Bookſellers, and to ſearch every Library where there was any Probability of its being lodged; and if his Enquiries ſhould prove unſucceſsful there, he was to proceed to* Italy, *and ſo on to other Countries till he ſhould find it. After a long and expenſive Search, he at laſt was ſo happy as to light upon two of them, which he purchas'd, tho' at an exorbitant Price, and brought them to his Noble Maſter, who was ſo pleaſed with the Purchaſe, that he not only paid him generouſly for his Time and Expences, but, over and above, as a Gratuity and Reward for his Diligence, preſented him with a Bank Note for* 30l.

Thus much for the Scarcity of the Book, it will in the next Place be proper to give ſome Account of the Subject of it, which is
S т о n e s,

STONES; *that is, all Manner of precious Stones that have been ever valued for their Beauty, Colour, Oddity, Curiofity, Ufe or Virtues, each of which the Author has fo exactly defcribed, and fo juftly affigned to its peculiar Stone, that it is almoft impoffible, for a Man of any tolerable Skill, to miftake the proper Name of a Stone at firft Sight, or not to know its Properties and Value.*

But tho' what I have faid, in regard to the Ufe and Excellence of this little Treatife, is inconteftibly the Truth; yet I muft give the Reader a Caution in the Perufal of it, which is this: That the Author living in an Age when Superftition univerfally prevail'd, and when the Study of Aftrology, Palmeftry, Charms, Spells, Sigils, &c. was greatly in Vogue, but which, in our Days, is entirely out of Ufe, at leaft is laid afide by the Learned: I fay, the Author, falling in with the Maxims of the Age wherein he lived, has affigned fuch Virtues to particular Stones as will

not

not be allowed by the *Moderns*; as that
such or such a *Stone* shall give the Pos-
sessor of it, *Courage*, procure him *Victory*
over his *Enemies*, make him successful in
Love, in *Litigations* at *Law*, and other
Undertakings, with other *Fancies* of the
same *Kind*, which have been long since ex-
ploded. He, however, gives us this *Caution*, that in his *Description* of the *Virtues* and *Properties* of *Stones*, he has in-
serted nothing but what he has collected
from the *Writings* of the most learned
Men that have treated of the *Subject*; so
that he exhibits nothing, or but very little,
as his own *Opinion*, nay, sometimes he ban-
ters and ridicules the extravagant *Fancies*
of those whose *Sentiments* he quotes: So
that when the *English* *Reader* meets with
these odd *Whimsies*, he is to look on them in
their proper *Light*, and to give a due *Attention* to the more weighty and important
Design, and *Use* of the *Book*.

The *Author* divides his *Treatise* into
three *Books*. In the *First*, he discourses

*philosophically on the Matter and Prin-
ciples of Stones, shews how and where they
are generated, from whence they derive
their various Beauties, Colours and Virtues, and gives such exact Rules for the
Knowledge of the True from the False and
Counterfeit, as must be extremely useful to
such as deal in this precious Commodity.*

*In the Second Book, he gives an alpha-
betical Description of all the various Stones
that have been ever taken Notice of by the
Learned and Curious, to the Number of
two Hundred and upwards, and so minutely specifies their several Properties and
Attributes, that nothing is omitted that
may contribute to the perfect Knowledge of
any Stone that comes to Hand.*

*The Third Book we have wholly omitted,
for the Reasons following. The Author
there treats of the Sculpture on Stones engraved by the Antients, but says, there are
few who understand the Import of these
Seals and Impressions on Stones, unless they*

at the same Time are skill'd in the Astro-
nomical, Magical and Necromantic Sci-
ences.   He then gives an Account of those
Sculptors among the Antients who were
most famous in this Art, that the Israel-
ites, *while in the Wilderness, were the*
First who distinguished themselves by these
Kinds of Works, and that the antient Romans *were the greatest Artists in this*
Way, and after he has given a List of the
most famous Sculptors among the Antients,
and of those who flourish'd in his own
Time, he proceeds to shew the particular
Virtue of an engraved Stone, how it re-
ceives that Virtue, and how it commu-
nicates it, according to the Nature and
Difference of the Image or Figure impress'd
on it ; gives Reasons why Stones engraven
have more Virtue in them than those that
are not so ; in what Manner Stones imbibe
the Influence of the Planets and Constella-
tions, why a Stone engraven with any of
the Twelve Signs of the Zodiac, is suppo-
sed to take its Virtue from that Sign, and
what its peculiar Virtue is.   He likewise
gives

gives us many Particulars of the same Nature, from the Works of Salomon, a famous Magician, and from the Writings of Hermes, a noted Astrologer. But as nothing of this Kind suits the Taste of the more enlighten'd Moderns, we judged it wholly impertinent to trouble our Readers with Speculations not agreeable to right Reason, nor indeed consistent with our Religion However, if the Curious, for their Amusement, are desirous of knowing the Sentiments of the Antients in these Matters, upon the Intimation of their Desire, we will give them a Translation of this our Author's Third Book, in a small Volume by itself.

As to the Author, CAMILLUS LEONARDUS, I can give no other Account of him than what is to be gather'd out of this little Piece; namely, that he was a Physician of some Eminence in the antient City of Pisaro in Italy, and that he was high in the Esteem of CÆSAR BORGIA, to whom he dedicates this Treatise : That he

was

was a learned Man, and well acquainted with Authors, may eaſily be diſcern'd by his Manner of treating the Subject he has here taken in Hand. But I ſhall detain the Reader no longer from a more agreeable Amuſement.

THE

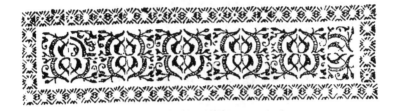

THE
PROEMIUM.

ALtho᷐ many learned Men, both antient and modern, have wrote upon
Stones, yet none of them have given
ns a complete Treatife on the Subject. My
Purpofe therefore, in this little Book, is to
treat minutely of Stones. For in Stones there
are many Things to be confider'd with refpect to their Effence. As firft, the Matter;
alfo, their Virtues, then the Images imprefs'd
on them. Therefore this Book, which is en-
titled the MIRROR OF STONES, will be divided into three Books. Alfo, the Name of
it, the MIRROR, is given it for a like Reafon, viz. that as a *Mirror*, or Looking-
glafs, truly reprefents the Images of Things
fet before it; fo in this Book, all thofe Things
which

which can reasonably be made the Subject of Enquiry in relation to Stones, are set in their proper Light.

The First Book.

CHAP. I.

Of the Matter of Mixts, but principally of Stones.

ALL the Philosophers, most Illustrious and Mighty *Cæsar*, are perfectly clear in this, that all Things produced by Nature, which exist under the Orb of the Moon, are compounded of the Four Elements, and that according to their Specifick Qualities, they, more or less, partake of and derive their Virtues from these four Elements. This in particular is the Sentiment of that consummate Philosopher *Aristotle*, who, in his *third Book of Heaven and the World*, has these precise Words, " The Elements are the first Bodies, " from which other Bodies are made " Also, in his second Book *of Generation and Corruption*, " It is necessary that mixed Bodies should " consist of all the Elements, and not of one only "

only." This is likewife the Opinion of that moft illuftrious Prince of Phyficians, *Avicen*, where he fays: " The Elements are Bodies, and " the firft Parts of the Human Body, and of " other Things which cannot be divided into " Bodies of divers Forms, from whofe Com- " mixture are produc'd divers Species of Ge- " neration." From thefe and many other Au- thorities, which at prefent muft be omitted, it may be concluded, that the Elements are the Things which concur in and give Being to the Mixed or Compofite · But in what Manner they concur in giving Being to the Mix- ed, would be a too long, and ufelefs Enquiry ; fince it has been often handled by Phyficians, and efpecially by the *Conciliator*, in his 16th Difference. And when the two Elements, namely, Earth and Water, feem to have a greater Corpoieity or Denfity than the other two Elements , then we fay, that the Mixed abound more with thefe than with the reft. But as Minerals are of two Sorts, fome flux- ible or liquifiable, and others not , we fay, that the fluxible or liquifiable abound more with the Aqueous, as Metals , agreeable to the Opinion of *Ariftotle* in his fourth Book *of Meteors*. But Stones are not fluxible, altho' they abound with Water, becaufe of the Commixture of their dry Terrene , and there-

B   fore

fore dismissing the first Fluxibles, such as
Gold, Silver, and the like, our Discourse
shall be only on Stones: And for our principal Foundation we shall adduce the Authority of the great Prince of Philosophers, who,
in his Book of *Minerals*, says: " The Principles therefore of Stones are either of a
clayey and unctuous Substance; or of a Substance in which Water is most prevalent " By
clayey Substance we are to understand the
Earth   Neither shall we depart from the
Authority of that consummate Philosopher
Albertus Magnus in his Book *of Minerals*,
who holds, that Stones are of a double
Kind, and saith, that some abound with an
Aqueous, mix'd with a Terrene Dry, as
Chrystal, Beril, and the like, and others
with a dry Aqueous, but more of the Terrene, as Marble, Jasper, and the like   But
those which abound most with the Aqueous
and the Terrene Dry, are properly called Gems,
from the *Greek* Word, *gemma*, which in *Latin*, signifies to shine, for all such Stones are
glittering   Some, as I before observed,
abound with a dry Terrene, do not li-
quify, and also sink in Water.   For if they
were freed from that dry Terrene, they would
swim in Water, and melt like Ice   For there
is no Stone but will, by Reason of its Earthi-
ness.

nefs, fink in Water, fo it be not porous or full of Air. But Stones which abound moftly with the Terrene, are thick and dark, neither are thefe free from Water, according to *Ariftotle* in his Book of Minerals above cited, who expiefly fays. " Pure Earth " doth not become a Stone, becaufe it makes " no Continuation, but a Brittlenefs; the " prevalent Drinefs in it permits it not to con- " glutinate, and fo by the Aqueous mixed " with the Terrene, Stones are made." By the Aqueous he underftands an unctuous or vifcous Humidity, propoitioned with a Terrene affifted with a drying Heat. And according to the Proportion or Difpofition of fuch Humidity with the dry Terrene, divers and various Stones are produced For it often happens that this Humidity is not fo much or fo fubtil as that it can flow to all the Parts of the Earth itfelf; from which Deficiency it proceeds, that that Part of the Earth is not turned into a Stone. And this is the Reafon, that in Quarries of Stones there is found between the Stones a very thick Earth, which occafions a Difcontinuation of the Stones For if there was a fufficient and proportionate Humidity, the whole Stone would be continuous, as in many Places we fee Mountains of one Stone. And it often happens that

B 2   fuch

fuch Humidity is difproportioned by the Fluxi-
bility, altho' in Quantity it be fufficient, and
therefore it refides more in one Part than in
another, and when it is there condens'd by
the Heat, it produces a Sort of Knottinefs
in the Stones. And hence it is that Knots appear in Stones, as there are fome in your
Highnefs's Mountains, which Knots, by
Reafon of their great Humidity, can hardly
be cut or broken, as it is in other Stones
which abound with the Aqueous Here then
we fhall put an End to this Chapter, and conclude, that the Matter of Stones is the very
Elements, and as we have faid, in fome the
Aqueous with the dry Terrene moft abounds,
and in others the Terrene with an Aqueous
Humidity, yet not fo as wholly to difcharge
thofe Stones from other Elements; as we
fhall explain in the fixth Chapter, when we
come to treat of the Colour of Stones.

C H A P.

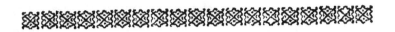

CHAP. II.
Of the effective or generative Cause of Stones.

THE effective or generative Caufe of Stones is by many diverfly affign'd. But, omitting vain Opinions, let us proceed to the true Caufe. We will affirm then, with the greateft Philofophers, that the effective or generative Caufe of Stones, is a certain Mineral Virtue, which not only exifts in Stones, but in Metals, and alfo in Things of a middle Nature between both · But as we want a proper Name for this Virtue, the Philofophers themfelves have invented one, that is, *the Mineral Virtue*; for what we cannot explain by proper Names fhould be illuftrated by fomething fimilar. Not that Examples can exactly fhew in what Manner this Mineral Virtue exifts in Stones, fays *Ariftotle*, for we do not give an Example that the Thing is fo, but that Learners may underftand; and fo by an Example which we fhall bring from the Animal Seed, it will appear, in what Manner the Mineral Virtue, which we fay is

effective

effective or generative, operates in Stones
Thus we fay, that the Seed of an Animal, is
a fuperfluous Nutriment defcending to the
Spermatick Veffels, and proceeding from
thofe Veffels The effective or generative
Virtue is infufed into the Seed itfelf, by the
Affiftance of which, the Spermatick Matter
is render'd prolific, as it is held in Phyficks.
Which Virtue however does not act by the
Mode of Effence, but by the Mode of Inhe-
rence Thus we fay, the Artificer is in the
Thing which is made by his Art In like
Manner we fay, that in apt Matter, in the Production of a Stone, there is the forming or
efficient Virtue in the producing of a Stone of
this or that Species, according to the Difpofition or Exigence of the Matter, and of the
Place and Influx, where fuch prepared Matter is found Which Virtue is indeed called
by fome, *the Celeftial Virtue*. And this is the
Meaning of *Plato*, where he fays, that the
Celeftial Virtues are infufed according to the
Goodnefs of the Matter. In Phyficks alfo it
is fhewn, that every Virtue forming and af-
fecting fomething in any Species, has its proper Inftrument, by Means of which it effects
or produces its Operation. Hence we fhall
follow the Opinion of *Ariftotle*, in his Book
of Minerals, and affert, that the proper effective

tive or generative Virtue of Stones, exifting
in the Matter of Stones, and is called Mineral, is conftituted of two Inftruments, which
Inftruments are diverfified according to the
Diverfity of the Nature or Species of
Stones. Of which Inftruments, the one is hot,
digeftive, and extractive or drying of the
Humid, inducing the Form of the Stone by
the Help of terreftrial Coagulation, which is
caufed by the unctuous Humid, and this
Heat is directed by the forming or Mineral Virtue of the Stones, which *Ariftotle* calls
the hot and drying Caufe. And there is
no Doubt, that if fuch Heat fhould not
be regular, but fhould exceed the Nature of
the Stone, it would crumble to Duft ; and if it
fhould be too fmall, it would not digeft well,
and fo could not bring that Matter into the
beft and perfect Form of a Stone. The other
Inftrument is a frigid Conftrictive in the Matter of the humid Aqueous, which humid A-
queous is fpread out by the dry Terreftrial ;
and this is the frigid Conftrictive of the
Humid, which Humidity, by the Intervention of fuch Conftriction, is preffed out, nor
does more remain in the Matter than is required for its Continuation, and this *Ariftotle*
calls the drying and congealing Virtue of the
Earth. And this is the Reafon that Stones

can by no Means be diffolved by a hot Drinefs, as Metals are melted   For in Metals
fuch Humidity is not wholly prefs'd out,
by Means of which, the Matter of the fluxible
Metal remains   Therefore we fay, that the
hot, digeftive and extractive Part of the Humid, and the frigid conftrictive Part of the
Humid, diffufed by the dry Terreftrial,
are the proper Inftruments of the formative or
Mineral Virtue of Stones.   And this is what
Ariftotle fays in his Book of *Minerals*, that
Stones are made two Ways, either by Conge-
lation or Conglutination ; as has been before
mentioned.

CHAP. III.

Of the fubftantial Form of Stones.

OF the fubftantial Form of Stones we
fhall not fay much in this Chapter,
as it will be more properly referved for the
Beginning of the fecond Book , where we
fhall fhew in what Manner Virtues are in
Stones, fince the fubftantial Form is that
which gives to Stones their Specifick Quality,
and from which very Virtue we may fay they
flow ,

flow; and therefore at prefent we fhall only deliver a philofophic Opinion. We fay then, that the fubftantial Form of a Stone is the Specifick Effence of that Stone ; which Effence comes from the Commixture of Elements, with a certain Proportion which leads to a determinate Species and to no other, by the Intervention of which, as we fhall fhew in the fecond Book, Virtues are in Stones. Nor does fuch Form proceed entirely from the Matter, nor is it placed wholly without the Matter : But it is fomething Divine above the complectionate Matter into which it is infufed, and below the celeftial Virtues by which it is given. This then we affert, that fubftantial Form is the fimple Effence of the Stone itfelf, by Means of which the Virtues of Stones are made to appear, which Virtues are varied not only in the different Species of Stones, but alfo in one Species, either by Reafon of the Place of their Generation, or of the Purity or Impurity of the Matter , as it happens in living Creatures.

C H A P.

✱✱✱✱✱✱✱✱✱✱✱✱✱✱✱✱✱

CHAP. IV.

Of the Place of the Generation of Stones.

SInce Place muſt neceſſarily concur in the Generation of all Things, and without which nothing can be generated or exiſt ; we ſhall therefore now diſcourſe of the Place of the Generation of Stones. Places not only diſtinguiſh the Diverſity of Species, but very often cauſe a Variety in one and the ſame Species ; as may be collected fiom the Diſcourſe of *Hermes,* who ſays, that Stones of the ſame Species, are varied in Power, as alſo in their Matter, by the Diverſity of Places ; meaning nothing moie by the Climate, than the different Direction oi Obliquity of the Rays of the Stais, which have Influence on inferior Things. We may aſſert then, that no determinate Place is appropriated to the Generation of Stones , ſince in almoſt every Part of the Eaith, Stones divers and various aie generated. Neither is there a proper Place aſſigned for it in a particular Element ; foi ſometimes we ſee them generated in the Earth, ſometimes in the Water, and ſome-

tinies

times in divers Places, as *Salomon* affirms in
his Book *of precious Stones*, where he says,
that there are divers Kinds of Stones and generated in divers Places; for some are found in
the Sea, others in different Parts of the Earth,
others in Rivers, others in the Nests of Birds,
some in the Intrails of Animals, some in the
Heads of others, others in the Reins of Dragons, Serpents, Beasts and Reptiles And
not only in such Places are Stones generated,
but, as Philosophers hold, even in the Air,
but especially that consummate Philosopher, and my most worthy Master, *Gaetane*
of *Fiena*, in his Comment of Meteors, in the
End of the second Treatise of the third Book;
where he says, Stones may be generated in
the Air, when an Exhalation has gross terrene Parts mixed with a gross and viscous
Humidity, and its more subtil Parts being
resolved, and the Terrestrial condensed by the
Heat, it becomes a Stone, which by its Gravity descends to the Earth. In our Times, a
huge Stone fell from the Clouds in *Lombardy*.
Pliny also in his first Book, Chap 60 writes,
that *Anaxagoras* foretold that a Stone would
fall from the Sun, which accordingly fell in
a Part of *Thrace* by the River *Egos*, of the
Bigness of a Cart, and of an adust or burnt
Colour. Nor do I wonder at this, since *Ari-*
stotle

ftotle affirms in his Book of Minerals, that a Piece of Iron of confiderable Magnitude fell out of the Air. But fince in Phyficks it has been determin'd, that the Stars, by their Quantity, Light, Motion and Situation govein the inferior World, according as every Matter is generative or corruptible; and as this Virtue of the Stars is ftrong throughout the World, wherefoever therefore an apt Matter is found, there will be the Place for the Generation of a Stone; fo that the proper and determinate Place for the Generation of a Stone is not to be affigned. It is neceffary however, that the Virtue of the Place in the Generation of a Stone fhould be diftinguifhed into three Virtues. Of which the firft is, the Virtue of the Mover moving the Orb; the fecond is the Virtue of the Orb moved, which Virtue is to be confidered many Ways in refpect to the Orb itfelf, as in the Planets and all the Conftellations The third is the Elementary Virtue, which is hot, frigid, humid and diy, or a Mixture of all thefe. The firft Virtue is as Form directing and forming every Thing that is generated, which Viitue, for Inftance, is brought upon thefe fenfible inferior Things, as the Virtue of an Art upon the Matter of Workmanfhip. The fecond is brought in as the Operation of an Inftrument

which

which is moved and directed by the Hand of
the Workman, in order to perfect the Work
begun. And this is that which *Ariſtotle* ſays,
that the Work of Nature is the Work of the
Underſtanding. Hence we ſay, that in whatever Place the unctuous Earth is mixed by the
Vapour reflected into itſelf, or where the
Strength of the Earth ſhall ſeize the Nature of
the Water, and draw and ſtrongly incline it
to a Drineſs, there undoubtedly is the Place of
the Generation of Stones. We may therefore
conclude and aſſert, that the Place proper and
fitteſt for the Generation of Stones, is an Earth
having a denſe Surface with a moderate Humidity, thro' which Denſity the Vapour cannot exhale. But the Earth that is thin, ſandy
and muddy, is of a contrary Temper; and
tho' Stones may be generated in ſuch Places,
yet they are imperfect. Very often alſo there
is in Water the greateſt Virtue in producing
Stones; not that Water is the beſt adapted
for it; but when it runs thro' mineral
Places, it aſſumes the Nature of thoſe Mines,
as we ſee the Waters of Baths acquire Heat
And when it is poured upon the Earth, or
any Thing is put into it, it ſeems to turn to
a Stone, as *Albertus Magnus* relates, and as
evidently appears in the Places of the Baths
where all Things ſeem as if they were petrified,

fied, and are continually augmented. This
is likewise the Sense of *Aristotle*, in his Book
of *Minerals*, that Water becomes Earth,
when the Qualities of the Earth overcome
the Water, and on the contrary, of Water is
made Earth. But we need not fetch Examples so far · Does not this manifestly appear,
Great *Cæsar*, near your own City, in the *Ca-
priolian* Fountain, where by the Course of its
Water, which has a Mineral in it, all the Ca-
nals are so petrified, and so incumber'd, that
the Water wants a Current ? *Aristotle* also,
in his said Book of *Minerals*, affirms, that
the Strength of the Mineral Virtue is sometimes so great, that it turns Water into Stone,
and every Thing contained in it ; from
whence it sometimes happens, that in many
Stones there are distinctly seen Parts of
aquatic Animals, and other Things turned
into Stone. Much might be said on this
Head, since Things have been found sometimes in the Earth, sometimes in the Water,
that have been petrified. *Albertus* gives an
Account of a Tree found on the Shore of the
Lucan Sea, with a Nest and Birds petrified

C H A P.

✿✿✿✿✿✿✿✿✿✿✿✿✿|✿✿✿✿✿✿✿✿✿✿✿✿✿

CHAP. V.

Of the Accidents of Stones, and first of their bad or good Composition.

AS in the former Chapters we have treated of those Things which contribute to the Generation of Stones, such as the Matter, the Efficient, the substantial Form, and the Place of Generation itself; now, to finish those Things which contribute to the Existence of Stones, it is Time to enquire about their Accidents, for even Accidents help to the Knowledge of the Subject in which they are placed, as *Aristotle* holds in his first Book *of the Soul.* But since those Accidents in Stones are many, our Discourse, for the present, shall be only of their good or bad Commixture, which in Stones happens many Ways. For a bad Commixture, or that which makes a Stone bad, sometimes happens by Reason of the Humid, sometimes by the Abundance of the Terrene, sometimes from the Indisposition of the hot or cold Agent, and sometimes from the Unfitness of the Piece, which gives a Diversity to Stones.

For if the Earth fhould be dry, it would be but badly commixed with the Humid, nor would be in a fufficient Quantity, and the Place wherein was fuch Matter for the producing fuch Stones, would be porous ; then the Heat, neceffary for the Being of the Stone, introduc'd by the effective Virtue, would evaporate, and fo could not well digeft the Parts of the Earth, and be mixed with the Humid ; whereby fuch a Stone would become fandy and gravelly, fo that it might be eafily filed, and reduc'd to Gravel. But if fuch a Place fhould not be porous, and fhould retain a temperate Heat with a fufficient Humidity, then a Stone produc'd of fuch an Earth would become hard, not liable to be broke into Sands, tho' it fhould appear gravelly, as is manifeft in the Porphyry Flint and others ; for in thofe Stones there are feen as it were little Sands, and are varied and diverfified in Bignefs and Colour, according to the Diverfity of the Drinefs of the Earth and of the acting Heat And fo fuch Heat exceeding the Humid, would burn the Parts of that Earth , in which Cafe the Stones would be difcontinuous, and appear like little Stones. But if in fuch a dry Earth the vifcous Humidity were imbibed, and confequently not fluxible, altho' it fhould have a regular

Heat

Heat from the mineral Virtue, and fhould be in a fit Place for the Generation of a Stone, it would not become united and continuous, but would be divided into little Stones of different Quantities and Colours, according to the Diverfity of the Matter concurring to the Effence of thofe Stones. But if fuch Humidity fhould be in Part fluxible and govern'd by a regular Heat, and in a proper Place, and be partly vifcous, a Stone would be formed of divers Colours and Parts with a Continuity, as tho' fuch Stones were joined with a Glew, as is feen in many Places, at *Venice*, in the Church of the Protector of that City, at *Rome* in many Places, and in the Door of your Highnefs's Study, and in cut Pillars in many Places, in which appear Colours fo various and divers, and fuch a wonderful Variety of Things, as hereafter fhall be declared. But the beft Commixture of Stones is made by Oppofition in the Things aforefaid, namely, that the Matter be not very dry, that the Humid be proportionate and fluid to every Part of the Earth, and that the Heat be proportion'd and regulated by the mineral or effective Virtue of the Stone itfelf, and that it be in a congruous and fitting Place, in Solidity and Rarity; all which being thus difpofed render Stones

C   uniform

uniform, even, and of the beſt Compoſition, and very often ſhining, according to the Commixture or Proportion of Earth and Water. But the oppoſite Cauſes, from the Things aforeſaid, make an Oppoſite. But that the Stone ſhould be very perfect, there is required a proportionate Heat, ſince that is the principal Agent, and by Means whereof a Diverſity is produc'd in Stones, and eſpecially in thoſe in whoſe principal Matter the Terrene is predominant. But in Stones which abound with the Aqueous, as its principal Matter, there are not ſo many Diverſities, ſince they have for their effective Virtue a frigid and dry Terrene. For the Parts of ſuch, by Reaſon of their Aquoſity, are well intermixed together, as the Fluxibles are diſtributed to every Part ; and therefore ſuch Stones obtain a good Degree of Perſpicuity and Hardneſs.

C H A P

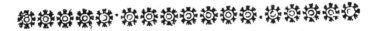

CHAP. VI.

Of the Perspicuity and Opacity of Stones, and of their Colour.

PErspicuity, or Opacity, occasion many Differences in Stones, since by Means of these, they may appear in the Colours themselves, as, according to the Philosopher, is held of the Sense and Things sensible, when he says, that Colour is the Extremity of the Perspicuous in a terminate Body. As also by the Commentator *Avenroes*, who holds, that Colour arises from the Commixture of a lucid Body with a dark Therefore before we ascertain some Differences about the Accidents in the Colour of Stones, it is necessary to declare in what Manner Perspicuity or Opacity happens in Stones, and what one and the other really is. We assert then, that Perspicuity is the material Existence of a Stone with a Transparency, or a kind of Brightness, and Opacity is accompanied with an Obscurity and Density. From whence it follows, that that Stone is perspicuous in whose Matter the more Causes of the Perspicuous concur, as Fire, Air, and Water; and, by Opposite, we say that

is

is opaque, in whofe Matter the opaque is moft prevalent, as is Earth. And when thefe Things are faid to terminate the Sight, which happens only from the Colour, it is neceffary to give them the Names of fome Colour, as we have before faid, which fhould be the terminative Colour of the Perfpicuous and Opaque, and fo, the Perfpicuous and Opaque are in the higheft Manner contrafted, and to them we attribute the Extremes of Colours For White is given to the Perfpicuous, and Black to the Opaque. Therefore we fay, the White is caufed by the Mixture of clear Fire with the Element which is very tranfparent, that is, the Air The Black is produc'd out of a turbid Fire mixed with the Element of the leaft Tranfparency, namely, the Earth But as thefe two Colours, the White and Black, are put for the Extremes, it is neceffary that they fhould partake of the intermediate Colours, and according to fuch Participation, great or lefs, arife divers Colours which are of a triple Kind, namely, Red, Green and Yellow And fo all Stones, exceeding the Extremes above-mention'd, are reduced to one of thefe, and are contained in them as the Species under its Genus But that we may attain to a perfect Knowledge of thefe Colours, it is neceffary to fhew how

those

thofe mediate Colours are caufed in Stones ;
and we fhall begin with the Red. The Red
Colour, we fay, happens in perfpicuous
Stones, when a lighted Fumofity and a
tender Fire is infufed in a perfpicuous Light ,
and all fuch Stones are faid to be glowing ,
of which Kind are all the Species of Carbuncles, as the *Balafius*, *Ruby*, *Jacinth*, &c.
which all agree in Rednefs, but differ according as they partake more or lefs of the Fire
of Fumofity and alfo of Perfpicuity. In the
fame Manner we may fpeak of the Yellow
perfpicuous Colour, whofe various Species
are produced, according to its fubtil and
perfpicuous Earthinefs, alter'd and burnt by
the Heat. But the Green is caufed by the
perfpicuous Aquofity with the burnt Terreftrial, which is diverfified in Stones, as it is
either aqueous or terrene, as in the two
mediate Colours above mention'd , from which
Diverfity the Green is varied, and various
green Colours are produc'd in Stones. Colours
alfo may be varied in the fame Stone, as in
the *Panther* and *Achates*, and many others ,
which Diverfity proceeds folely from the
Diverfity of the Subftance, or Matter which
concurs to its Exiftence Thus, as *Salomon*
in the fore-cited Place, fays, Colours are
diverfified in Stones, becaufe there is no

C 3   Colour

Colour to be found in Heaven, Air, Earth, Sea, Rivers, Herbs and Trees, which is not to be found in Stones. Many Things may be said of Colours, which for the Sake of Brevity, and that I may not tire the Reader, must be omitted; since what has been said of particular Colours, may lead us to the Knowledge of others. In such as are not perspicuous, the Whiteness is caused by the subtil Terrene mixed with the Aqueous. Blackness is occasion'd by a smoaky and aduſt Terrene, and in what Manner the Extremes of the Opaque, or not perspicuous Stones, seem to abound with much Earth, so also all the mediate Colours of those Opaque Stones, as the Red, Yellow and Green, seem to abound with much of the Terrene, as they participate the Nature of Extremes; which Terrene is compounded with the Igneous, Airy, and Aqueous in the Production of middle Colours, as we have said of the Perspicuous, that they abound with the Aqueous. But so it is that opaque Stones incline more or less to the perspicuous, as the Aqueous concurs more or less in their Composition, since these are the Things which give it Perspicuity. Likewise the Colours of those opaque Bodies are varied in one and the same Subſtance or Effence of the Stone

accord.

according to the Diverfity of the Parts com-
pofing that Stone, and alfo according to the
Power of the acting Heat, as we have faid
in the preceding Chapter.

CHAP. VII

Of the Hardnefs or Softnefs of Stones.

HArdnefs or Softnefs in Stones proceeds
from two Caufes; one of which
depends on the Matter of the Stone itfelf, the
other on the effective or mineral Virtues of
thofe Stones; as we have already faid in the
Chapter treating of the good or bad Mixture
of Stones. As to the Matter, we fay it
muft be well mixed, and it becomes fo by
the Aqueous, and therefore thofe Stones
which have the Aqueous predominant in
their Compofition, are the hardeft and moft
perfpicuous. Of this Sort are all thofe Gems
which refift the File, except the *Topaz*, as
we fhall fhew hereafter. But of thofe Stones
which in their Effence abound moft with the
Terrene, fome are hard and fome not, yet
are they not of that Hardnefs as the Aqueous, for the Reafon before given. Thofe

alfo

alſo are hard which abound with the Aqueous with a moderate Terrene; from which
Humidity altho' they may be opaque, yet
they have a lucid and a Sort of perſpicuous
Superficies, ſuch are the ſerpentine Porphyry,
and the like, and which can hardly be cut
aſunder with Iron, and ſcarcely with Steel.
But thoſe which abound with the Terrene
without a moderate Humid, are tender.
They likewiſe become tender and hard, as
the effective Virtue prevails. For when that
Virtue is not proportion'd to the Matter in
drying the ſuperfluous Humidity, they are
not render'd hard, ſince Hardneſs proceeds
from a temperate Drineſs, as all Phyſicians
hold. And therefore, as we have and do
affirm, the *Topaz* is not hard, as its effective
Virtue is deficient in Drineſs, nor can enough
abſorb the Humidity, of which a great deal
of ſuperfluous remains in it, and by Means
of which it is hinder'd from becoming hard.
What has been ſaid of the *Topaz* may be
affirm'd of all other Stones, which for their
effective Virtue, have their Heat and Drineſs diminiſhed We might enlarge on this
Head, but ſhall here end it, by aſſerting,
that Hardneſs proceeds from a temperate
Dryneſs, which ought to be regulated by
the effective Virtue, together with a good

Diſpo-

Difpofition of the Matter and Place, as wer obferv'd in the Fifth Chapter. From which Things being oppos'd, many Accidents happen in Stones, for fome refift the Fire, others are confumed by it, fome are fplit by the Froft, and reduc'd to Afhes, fome harden'd by the Air, others deftroyed by it The like and other different Accidents happen to Stones, both from the Water and the Sun, and from extrinfic Alterants, the Caufes of which it would be ufelefs here to enarrate, and may be eafily comprehended from what has been before and fhall hereafter be faid, efpecially by fuch as are of a clear Underftanding, fince all thefe Things confift in a fantaftical and imaginary Virtue.

C H A P. VIII.

Of the Gravity and Lightnefs, Denfity and Porofity of Stones.

GRavity or Lightnefs are Accidents proceeding from two Caufes in Stones. One of which is derived from a bad Compofition, an Accident which thofe Stones

are

are chiefly liable to whofe Subftance is terrene, and is occafion'd by a bad Mixture
of the Parts of the Earth reciprocally with
the Water. For when thofe aqueous Parts
are dried up by the effective Virtue, or thofe
which were not well mixed with the Earth
are diffolved, there remain Porofities in
thofe Stones, from whence they become
light. This Accident may likewife befal
Stones, from a Concurrence of too great a
Quantity of Air or Fire in the Subftance of
the Stone, and this Lightnefs accruing in
this Manner, is lefs frequent in opaque than
in perfpicuous Stones, but only the firft
Gravity in the opaque, proceeds from the
aforefaid contrary Caufes However, there
is never naturally fuch a Lightnefs in Stones,
but from their own Terreftcity they will fink
in Water, which indeed is the Property of a
Stone And altho' fome Sorts of Wood are
heavier than Stones, yet do they not fink in
Water as Stones do, the Reafon of which is,
that the material Subftance of the Wood has
not fo much of the dry Terrene In like
Manner we may affirm, that Denfity or Po-
rofity proceeds from the fame Caufes as do
Lightnefs or Gravity. But altho' many
other Accidents may happen, yet thefe fhall
fuffice for the prefent, fince from what has
been

been already faid, and is yet to be declared,
we may be able to affign a Caufe for all
the Accidents that may happen in them, and
efpecially may thofe who are fkill'd in Phyfick know them, fince thefe Things depend
on that Art.

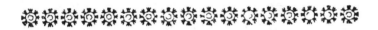

C H A P. IX.

*How to know whether Jewels are natural
or artificial.*

SInce thefe Times abound with Counterfeits in every Thing, but efpecially in the
Jewelling Art in regard to their Value ; and
as there are few, unlefs fuch as have been
long practis'd in them, can judge of them,
efpecially when they are cemented together ;
and that we may not be deceived by thefe,
nor leave any Thing untouch'd relating to
the Subject, we fhall clofe the Firft Book
with a few Things upon this Head. We
fay then, that thefe deceitful Artifts in Stones
have many Ways of Impofition. As firft,
when they make Stones of a lefs Value, and
of a particular Species, appear of another
Species

Species and confequently of a higher Price;
as the *Balafius* of the *Amethift*, which they
perforate, and fill the Hole with a Tincture,
or bind it with a Ring, or more fubtilly, when
they work up the Leaves of the *Balafius*,
either with *Citron Saphire* or *Beril*, into the
Form of Diamonds, and by adding a Tincture
to bind them, fell them for true Diamond.
Or, very often they fabricate the upper
Superficies of the *Granate*, and the lower of
Chryftal, which they cement with a certain
Glew or Tincture, fo that when they are
fet in Rings they appear like *Rubies* And
many other Deceptions may be effected out
of divers and various Stones, which are all
known to the Skilful.   Therefore, when
there is a Sufpicion, the Jewels are to be
taken out of the Rings, and by what we
have farther to fay in the Second Book, we
may eafily judge of them.   A Deception
may happen in another Manner, as when
they make the Form and Colour of a true
Stone from one that is not true.   And this
Deception is made from many Things, and
chiefly from fmelted Glafs, or of a certain
Stone, with which our Glafs-makers whiten
their Veffels, by adding divers permanent
Colours to the Fire, as the Potters know,

and

and as I have often feen *Emeralds,* far
from bad ones, at leaft for Ufe, made out
of thefe Stones Thefe counterfeit Stones
may be known many Ways, as firft by the
File, to which all falfe Stones give Way,
and all natural ones are Proof againft, except
the *Emerald* and the Weftern *Topaz,* as we
fhall fhew in the Second Book, and therefore thefe Falfifiers chufe to work upon thefe
which give way to the File, becaufe they
cannot be prov'd by it. The fecond Way
to prove them is by the Afpect; for fuch
as are natural, the more they are look'd at,
the more the Eye is delighted with them ;
and when they are held up to the Light of
the Candle, they fhine and look fulgent
Whereas the Non-naturals, or artificial, the
more they are beheld, the more the Sight is
wearied and difpleas'd, and their Splendor
feems continually decaying, efpecially when
they are oppos'd to the Light of a Candle.
They are alfo known by their Weight when
they are out of the Rings, for thofe which
are natural are ponderous, except the Emerald, but the Artificial are light. There is
one Proof yet remaining, which is infallible,
and is prefeable to all the reft, namely, that
the Artificial do not refift the Fire. but are
liqui-

liquified in it, and lose their Colour and Form when they are diffolved by the Fiercenefs of the Fire; and it is impoffible but that in fome Parts of them, fome Points like fmall Bubbles muft be feen in their Subftance, produc'd by the igneous Heat, and will difcover the Difproportion in their Compofition, and their Difference from Nature in true Stones. Such falfe Stones may likewife be compounded of other Things than of Glafs, namely, of many Minerals; as of Salt, Copperas, Metals, and other Things, and as I have feen, and is allowed by many learned Men, efpecially by Brother *Bonaventure* in the Second Book of his Dictionary of Words, that the Knowledge of Stones, and their Species, is acquired by great Experience, and from continual Ufes, as they well know who employ themfelves in this Kind of Exercife. And here we fhall conclude this firft Book.

BOOK

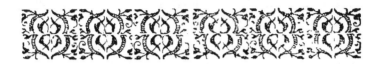

BOOK II.

CHAP. I.

The Proem.

HAVING, moſt Illuſtrious Prince, finiſhed the Firſt Part of my Work, wherein I have, in general treated of the Generation of Stones, and their Accidents ; I ſhall now, in this ſecond Book, ſpeak particularly of the Stones themſelves. The firſt Argument ſhall be, whether there be Virtue in Stones, and in what Manner they communicate their Virtues to us, by alledging the Opinions of the Antients, with the true Judgment of Philoſophers. I ſhall likewiſe give the Names of thoſe learned Men from whoſe Works I have compiled this Tract, that the Reader may be ſatisfied that what I have wrote, is taken from them. I ſhall give the Names of all Stones, in the Order of the Alphabet, together with their

Colours,

Colours, the Places where they are found and their Virtues where any are afcribed to them by the Learned.

❋❋❋❋❋❋❋❋❋❋❋❋|❋❋❋❋❋❋❋❋❋❋❋

C H A P. II.

Whether there be Virtues in Stones, with the various Opinions concerning the fame.

THere is no fmall nor ufelefs Contention among the moft celebrated Doctors concerning the Virtues of Stones. Some of them fay there is no Virtue in Stones, which we think is falfe, and therefore fhall difmifs them as wholly deviating from the Truth. There are others who fay, there is only an Elementary Virtue in Stones, fuch as Heat, Cold, Hardnefs, Paffibility, and the like, which are inherent to their Compofition, and proceed from the elementary Effence, but deny all other Virtues arifing from the Specific Form or Subftantial Effence of the Stone; fuch as to difpel Poifons, obtain Victory, and the like And this is their trifling Way of Reafoning Thofe Things, fay they, which are of a nobler Kind, ought

to

to have in them the nobler Virtues. But as Things animate are more noble than those which are inanimate, therefore the more noble Virtues might be expected in the Animate, rather than in the Inanimate, but as the Animate want those Virtues, therefore so do Stones which are inanimate. They have likewise other perfuasive Reasons, which for Brevity's sake we omit. In the first Place, Experience itself is against these Gentlemen; for with our own Eyes we may see a Virtue in Stones. Don't we see the Magnet attract Iron? the Saphire cure Carbuncles, and the like in many others? A Man who should deny these Things could not be thought in his Senses, since they are known to us as first Principles. But farther, I will argue with these Disputants from a known Topick, thus: That which all Men proclaim for Truth, cannot be wholly groundless; but as it has been always allow'd, as well by some of the Antients as by all the Moderns, that there are Virtues in Stones, therefore we ought to give Credit to those learned Doctors who affirm it. The Authority of *Salomon* is of great Weight in this Matter, who says, That the Virtues of Stones are divers, some procure the Favour of Great Men, others are a Defence against Fire;

others

others render Perfons amiable; others give Wifdom, fome make Perfons invifible; fome repel Lightning; fome extinguifh Poifon; fome preferve and increafe Treafure; others influence Hufbands to love their Wives, fome quell Tempefts at Sea; others cure Difeafes, fome preferve the Head and Eyes. And, to conclude all, whatever can be thought of as beneficial to Mankind, may be confirmed to them by the Virtue of Stones: Yet this is to be noted, that in Stones there is fometimes one Virtue, fometimes two, fometimes three, and fometimes many; and that thefe Virtues are not caufed by the Beauty of the Stone, fince fome of them are moft unfightly, and yet have a great Virtue, and fometimes the moft beautiful have none at all, and therefore we may fafely conclude, with the moft famous Doctors, that there are Virtues in Stones, as well as in other Things; but how this is effected is varioufly contro- verted. It was one Opinion of the *Pytha- goreans*, that there were Virtues in all Things, communicated to them by the Soul, and that Stones and all inferior Things were animated, and faid, that Souls could enter into and depart from any Matter by the animal Operations, as the Human Under- ftanding extends itfelf to Things intelligible

and

and the Imagination to Things imaginable
Thus, fay they, it is in Stones, the Souls
of Stones extended themfelves from the
Place of the Stone's Refidence, to Man, and
fo imprefs'd its Virtue on the Subftance of
Man, and thus they held that Virtue was in
Stones, and that it operated by the Mediation
of the Soul, juft as Fafcination is wrought by
the Eye in the fame Way. They faid, that
the Soul of Man, or of any other Animal,
enter'd another Man or Animal by the Sight,
and hinder'd the Operation of that Animal;
which Fafcination, muft not be fuppos'd to
proceed folely from the Sight, fince Vifion
is effected by taking in, not by fending out
Of this Opinion *Virgil* feems to be in his
Bucolics, where he fays,

Nefcio quis teneros oculus mihi fafcinat agnos.

Such Kind of Fafcination is not peculiar
to Men, but is likewife feen in Brutes, as
both *Solinus* and *Pliny* affirm, nay, I myfelf
have obferv'd, that when the Wolves in
Italy face a Man, his Voice becomes
hoarfe, nor can they raife their Cry to fo
high a Tone, altho' before they had no Defect
in their vocal Inftrument. Nor does this
happen merely from the Sight, as before

D 2   hinted,

hinted, but from another Caufe, namely, from the Soul of the Fafcinator. *Demo-critus* follows this, who fays, that all Things are full of the Gods; alfo *Orpheus*, who fays, the Gods and divine Virtues are diffufed thro' all Things, and that nothing elfe was God but that which forms Things, and is diffufed through all Things, and fo imagin'd that the Gods were Souls, and attributed Virtue to Things by the Mediation of the Soul; which is falfe and abfurd, according to all Philofophers. But to pafs by thefe groundlefs Opinions, let us come to the Truth. But firft we fhall return an Anfwer to thofe contradicting Gentlemen above-mention'd To omit thofe who deny there is any Virtue in Stones, which is abfurd, and a Contradiction to all Philofophers, let us anfwer thofe who affirm, that there is only the Virtue of the Elements in Stones, when they fay, that the more noble Virtues ought to exift in Things which are more noble, &c. I grant that this is true, and fay, that in Things animate there are nobler Virtues than in Stones. Nobody in his Senfes doubts that in Man there are nobler Virtues than in Stones. But as to Brutes, thus much may be faid There are many Brutes in which we may difcover the Change of Time or Air,

as

as is held by many learned Men who have written of the Variation of the Air, particularly by that worthy Knight, Sir *Nicholas Patavinus*, the greateſt Aſtronomer of our Times, who aſſerts, that there are many Animals which foretel the Change of the Weather by their ſinging or aſſembling together. Do not Cocks, by their Crowing, diſtinguiſh the Hours of the Night? Which Animals not only demonſtrate a Virtue to be in ſuperior Things, but alſo have the greateſt in Things inferior, ſince from the Effects produc'd in them, we may infer there is the greateſt Virtue in Men, as we may learn from the Books of Phyſicians; all which Things I apprehend are much more noble than the Virtues of Stones. From which we ſhall conclude, that their Argument is groundleſs, and of no Force or Efficacy. To the third Diſputants, I ſhall only anſwer, that the Virtue of Stones does not proceed from the Soul, nor wholly from the Elements; but, as we ſhall hereafter explain the Matter, from the very Species or ſubſtantial Form of the Stone itſelf, as we ſhall evidently make appear from Opinions of Philoſophers.

D 3　　　　C H A P.

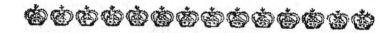

CHAP. III.

How, and from whence Stones have their Virtues.

TO return from this long Digreſſion; let us now come to the Matter in Hand. It is certain there are Virtues in Stones, but from whence they derive ſuch Kind of Virtue remains yet to be ſhewn. There are ſome who hold, that the ſpecial Virtues, as well as the complexional, in Stones, are from the Elements which compoſe them; and thus they reaſon. Whatever is compounded of any Thing, has the Virtue of the Thing compounding, as a Stream partakes of the Nature of the Fountain from whence it runs; but it is known that Stones are compounded of the Elements, as we have already declared; therefore whatever there is in Stones proceeds only from the Elements, and not from any other Virtue *Plato*, as likewiſe his Followers, who hold Ideas, ſay, that all compoſite Bodies, of whatever Species they are, have their Idea which infuſes Virtue into them, and by how much ſuch mixed or

com-

compofite Bodies partake of the purer Subftance of the Elements, by fo much does
their Idea, by the Mediation of the pure
Matter where it is infufed, induce a greater
Perfection.   Now, as precious Stones are of
this Sort, therefore their Idea produces a
greater Virtue in them, than in other compofite Bodies not fo pure ; and fo they
attribute fpecial Virtues to them by Means of
the interfering Idea.   *Hermes*, and other
Aftronomers, whofe Contemplations are
more exalted, fay, that the Virtues of all
inferior Things, proceed from the Stars and
the Figures in the Heavens.   And according
to which, as the Mixture is compounded of
the purer or groffer Elements, fo the Virtues
of the Stars, and the Figures of the Heavens,
communicate a greater or lefs Virtue   And
as precious Stones have the Purity of the
Elements, and, as it were, a Celeftial Compofition or Mixture, as in the *Saphire, Balafius,* and others , fo thofe Stones have a
greater Virtue than the reft of the Compofites,
which retain not fo much of the purer
Elements   Hence *Hermes*, concerning the
Caufe of the Virtue of Stones, faith, We
know for certain, that the Virtues of all
inferior Bodies defcend from the Superior ,
for the Superior by their Subftance, Light,

Situation and Motion, and also by their Figure, infuse all those noble Virtues which we find in Stones. It it plain therefore from what has been already said, as well as from the Opinion of *Ptolomy*, that the Virtues of Stones are derived from the Stars, the Planets, and the Constellations, thro' the affisting Purity of their own Complexion. Other Opinions might be alledged, but as they are frivolous, we shall not mention them, nor offer any more Arguments to confute those above-mention'd However none of those Opinions come nearer to the Truth than that of *Hermes*, and the rest of the Astronomers, who constantly affert, that inferior Bodies are govern'd by superior Influences; which is likewise the Judgment of all Philofophers.

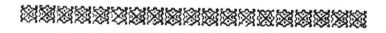

C H A P. IV.

Of the true Opinion of the Virtue of Stones.

BUT tho' the Opinions before alledg'd may have some Appearance of Truth, yet are they not Philofophical, for the

Philofopher holds, that Virtues proceed only
from the Form and Subftance of the Thing;
which is affirm'd by *Ariftotle* in his firft Book
of *Phyficks*, where he fays, That Matter
with Form is the Caufe of all Things, in
the Subject, juft as Matter or Subftance is
the Caufe of all Accidents *Albertus Magnus*,
who was a moft confummate Philofopher,
and a ftrict Obferver of Nature, is of
Opinion, that the Virtue of Stones comes
from the very Species and fubftantial Form
of the Stone itfelf. For in a mixed Body
there are fome Things, fuch as Hardnefs,
Gravity, and the like, whofe Caufe is the
Virtues of the Elements, and there are fome
Things whofe Virtues derive their Caufe
from the Species itfelf. For Example:
That the Magnet has Hardnefs, an iron
Colour, and the like, proceeds from the
Virtue of Mixtibles or the Elements; but
its attracting Iron proceeds from the Species
of the *Magnet* itfelf, which Species fhews us
an Aggregate of Form and Matter; according to the *Commentator*, in his firft Book of
Metaphyficks, where he declares, that Species
is not barely Form, but the whole Aggregate
of Form and Matter, which gives the indivi-
dual Eifence to this Matter. For the Effence
of all Things hath, according to its proper
Species,

Species, its Operation and peculiar Virtue,
according to the Species in which it is
form'd, and perfected in a natural Being.
And all complexionate Bodies are the Instru-
ments of their own Form; for the Form
ceasing, the Complexion is corrupted or
destroyed, so that Form is contain'd in the
Matter as its divine and most excellent Part.
For Form is something divine, below the
Celestial Virtues from whence it is deriv'd,
yet above the complexionate Matter into
which it is infused. So that Form is one
simple Essence, only operative of one Thing,
whatsoever it be, peculiar to its Species; for
one Thing can affect only one Thing, since
One is only productive of One. We may
likewise consider Form in another Light, as
a Celestial Virtue, which is multiplied in
inferior Things from the Images and Circles
of Heaven, which distribute Twelve Signs
with their Stars over the Horizon of the
Thing in which it is infused, and so
the Form is manifold according to the
elemental Virtues in which it is wrought, and
those natural Powers which contribute to its
simple Essence. Thus Form is productive
of many Effects, tho' perhaps it may have
only one proper Operation, and hence it is,
that almost all Things are not determin'd to

one

one Virtue only by its known Operations.
But only that Form which fpecifies the
Matter is more powerful than other Forms;
altho' very often the proper Form, from
the Indifpofition of the Matter, can be but
little fhewn or operate. Hence *Hermes*
fays, concerning Stones, that Stones of the
fame Species are varied in Power from
the Confufion of the Matter, alfo from the
Place of their Generation, thro' the Direct-
nefs or Obliquity of the Beams correfpond-
ing to thofe Places; fo that very often it
gives no peculiar Effect to its Species.
Wherefore, to confider it philofophically,
and with the Authority of *Albertus Magnus*,
we will venture to affirm, That the Virtues
of Stones proceed from the Species, by the
Mediation of the fubftantial Form of the
Stone itfelf, produc'd in a proper Place, and
of a proportionate Matter, adapted to the
Effence of fuch a Stone. This was likewife
the Opinion of *Plato*, who fays, that Nature has endowed fome Things with Properties, for every Thing has, in fome manner, that from its Species, which makes it
act that which is proper to it in its own
Species.

CHAP.

✿✿✿✿✿·✿✿✿✿✿✿✿·✿✿✿✿✿✿

CHAP. V.

*The Names of all those Learned Men,
whose Works have furnish'd us with
the Materials of the following Treatise.*

AS I am now to treat of particular
Stones, that I may not seem to advance any Thing on my own Authority,
I shall give a List of all those learned
Men, whose Works have assisted me on
this Occasion. But as I have found some
Disagreement between them, I shall only
adopt such Opinions, in which most of them
are agreed. Let Nobody therefore wonder,
if he should sometimes find me differing
from the Sentiments of some particular
Doctor, rather let him examine those whom
I name, before he passes too severe a Cen-
sure upon me, for he will find, that what
I shall advance is approved by the Majority
of them. And since I have undertook to
be a faithful Transcriber of the Sentiments of
all those learned Men who have wrote upon
this Subject, I will here give their Names·
viz.

viz. Dioſcorides ; Ariſtotle ; Hermes ; Evax ; Scapio ; Avicenna ; John Meſue ; Salomon ; Phyſiologos ; Pliny ; Solenus , Lapidaritus ; Heliamandus , Iſiodorus ; Arnaldus , Juba ; Dionyſius Alexandrinus , Albertus Magnus ; Vincentius the Hiſtorian ; *Thetel Rabanus ; Bartholomew of the Roman Rock ,* Biſhop *Marbodius , Ortulanus ;* the Book of the *Pandects , Cornucopiæ , Kirandus ,* and the Book *of the Nature of Things.* For, as I ſaid before, whoever well underſtands all the Writings of the Learned, will know, that I have not departed from thoſe Sentiments wherein the moſt of them are agreed, but have ſtuck cloſely to them , for I have taken all of them for my Guide in this little Treatiſe.

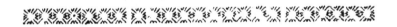

CHAP. VI

Of Particular Stones, in an Alphabetical Order.

THUS far, moſt Noble Prince, our Diſcourſe has been carried on in generals , we are now come to the Point which we had chiefly in View, that is, to ſpeak particularly of the Names and Virtues of

of Stones ; which fhall be the Bufinefs of
this whole Chapter according to the Order of
the Alphabet In the firft Place we fhall
give the proper Names of the Stones, and
add others if they have any, and from whence
they have them We fhall likewife defcribe
the Colour of Stones, and their Species, if
they have more than one, and in what Species the better Sort are contain'd ; to which
will be added the Place of their Generation
or Finding Laftly, as a Thing of much
more Value, and more defired by all, we
fhall defcribe their Virtues, that fo we may
acknowledge that all Things which have
been produc'd by the Supreme Artificer,
were defign'd for the Health or Welfare of
Mankind : To whom we ought to render
infinite Thanks, that he is not only careful
for the Welfare of the Soul, but likewife for
the Health of the Body.

A

Adamant, or the Diamond, is a moft precious Stone, of the Colour of polifh'd Iron,
and as it were Chriftalline. Its Quantity is
never found larger than the Bignefs of a
Filberd It will give way to no Sort of
Matter,

Matter, neither to Fire nor Iron, but defpifes all ; it had its Name from the *Greek* Interpretation, which is, *an unconquer'd Virtue*. Some hold, it can be mollified only by the warm Blood of a Goat, which is fabulous, fince I have feen many broke with the Blow of a Hammer. Neither is there any Thing fo hard, but it will fuffer by the *Adamant.* Strange it is, if the Report be true, that it is fuch an Enemy to the *Magnet,* that if it be bound to it, it will not attract Iron. Of this there are Six Species more particularly noted by the Learned, and named from the Places in which they are found, *viz* The *Indian, Arabick, Syrian, Macedonian, Ethicpick,* and the *Cyprian*, and of each in their Order. The *Indian* is fmall as to its Quantity, but excels in its Virtue, and this is that which refifts the Hammer ; it is ponderous, and of the Colour of a clear Chryftal The *Arabick* is like to this, but paler, and lefs in Quantity. The *Syrian* and *Macedonian* has the Colour of fhining Iron. The *Ethiopick* is the darkeft of all The *Cyprian* is of a Golden Hue, but bafer and fofter than all the reft. The Virtue of all thefe Species is to repel Poifon, tho' ever fo deadly ; is a Defence againft the Arts of Sorcery, difperfes vain Fears ; enables to quell all Quarrels

and

and Contentions; is a Help to Lunaticks, and such as are possess'd with the Devil; being bound to the left Arm, it gives Victory over Enemies; it tames wild Beasts; it helps those who are troubled with Phantasms, and the Night-mare, and makes him that wears it bold and daring in his Transactions. The *Indian* Adamant, and likewise the *Arabick*, has the Property of the *Magnet*, to direct the Needle touch'd by it to the Arctick Pole, and from hence some call it the Adamantine Loadstone.

Achates is a Stone of divers Colours, which are varied according to the Place of its Generation; of which there are many Species, but the most famous are these Seven, which, as Jewellers affirm, are not only varied in Colour, but even in their Virtue. *Sicily* gave the first *Achates*, which was found in the River *Acheus*. For which Reason the *Sicilian* is placed in the first Rank, then the *Cretian, Indian, Egyptian, Persian, Arabian*, and *Cyprian*. The *Sicilian* is black, intersected with a white Vein. *Crete* produces an *Achates* like a Filberd, with Gold Veins or Drops. The *Indian* is varied with many Colours and Veins, by the Intersection of which are often formed divers Figures; such as Wild Beasts, Flowers, Woods, and Birds, or

or fhews the natural Effigies of Kings, as in
that *Achates* of King *Pyrrhus*; and I have
feen an *Achates* in which appeared Seven
Trees ftanding on a Plain, and thefe are
univerfally efteemed the moft excellent. The
Egyptian wants Rednefs and Whitenefs, and
is interfected with various Veins. The
Perfian being heated, fmells like Myrrh, as
fome fay. *Dionyfius, of the Site of the World,*
affirms, that the *Perfian Achates* are in the
Form of a Cylinder, which being carried by
the Courfe of the Waters from the Tops of
the Mountains, are drove along the River
Coafpis, and are found among the Sands.
The *Arabian* and *Cyprian* are variegated with
divers Colours, tending to a glaffy Tranfparency. The Virtues of the *Achates* differ
according to the Diverfities of their Species;
but all of them agree in this, to make Men
folicitous. But the proper Virtue of the
Sicilian is, to fubdue the Poifon of Vipers
and Scorpions, if it be bound on the Punc-
ture, or being bruifed, drank in a Glafs of
Wine. The *Indian* is an Enemy to all venemous Things. It refrefhes the Sight by
looking on it. Being held in the Mouth it
quenches Thirft It gives Victory to him
that wears it, turns away Storms, and puts
a Stop to Lightnings. The *Cretan* fharpens

E   the

the Sight; extinguishes Thirst and Poisons;
renders the Wearer of it gracious and eloquent, and preserves and confirms Strength.
It seems superfluous to particularize the
Virtues of them all, since they coincide one
with another, and therefore, for Brevity's
Sake, we shall omit them.

Amethist, is reckon'd among the purple
and transparent Stones, mixed with a violet
Colour, emitting rosy Sparkles. Of which
there are five Species, but all of them bordering on the Purple, mingled with various
Colours. The *Indian* exceeds the others in
Colour, Beauty and Price, having a Purple
mixed with a rosy and midling Violet. But
those which are entirely Purple are not so
valuable as the Grape Violet, and the watery
Violet are baser than the rest. They are
denominated from the Places where they
are found. The *Indian* stands in the first
Rank. The *Arabian*, *Armenian*, *Galatian*,
Tarsian and *Cyprian*, follow in their Order;
tho' the two last are reckon'd baser than all
the rest, and of no Estimation, nor are they
taken any Notice of by the Learned. All
of them are fit for Engraving. Their Virtue
is to drive away Drunkenness, for being
bound on the Navel, they restrain the Vapour of the Wine, and so dissolve the

Ebriety,

Ebriety; they reprefs evil Thoughts, and give a good Underftanding, they make a Man vigilant and expert in Bufinefs, the Barren they render fruitful by drinking a Lotion of it, they expel Poifon, they preferve Military Men, and give them Victory over their Enemies, and prepare an eafy Capture of wild Beafts and Birds

Alectoria, is a Stone of a chriftalline Colour, a little darkifh, fomewhat refembling limpid Water, and fometimes it has Veins of the Colour of Flefh. Some call it *Gallinaceus,* from the Place of its Generation, the Inteftines of Capons, which were caftrated when they were three Years old, and had lived feven, before which Time it ought not to be taken out; for the older it is, fo much the better. When the Stone is become perfect in the Capon, he don't drink However, 'tis never found bigger than a large Bean The Virtue of this Stone is, to render him who carries it invifible, being held in the Mouth, it allays Thirft, and therefore is proper for Wreftlers, makes a Woman agreeable to her Hufband, beftows Honours, and preferves thofe already acquired, it frees fuch as are bewitched, it renders a Man eloquent, conftant, agreeable

E 2 and

and amiable, it helps to regain a loft Kingdom, and acquire a foreign one.

Androdamas, is an exceeding hard and heavy Stone like the *Adamant*, having the Brightnefs of polifh'd Silver. Its Figure is diftinguifhed into Squares or Dies, and is found among the Sands of the Red Sea. It's fuppos'd that it deriv'd its Name from its Virtue; which is to reftrain Anger and the violent Emotions of the Mind, alfo to mitigate Luxury and leffen the Gravity of the Body.

Aftroites, *Aftrion*, *Afterias*, or *Afterites*, is a white Stone approaching to Chriftal. It contains a Light like a Star included in it, moving from the Part where it receives the Light, when may be feen in it a Form like a Blazing Star, or burning Flame. It has its Name from *Aftrum*, that is, a Star, and not an Image. *Thrace* and *Carmenia* produce them, which being touch'd by the Solar Beams appear White.

Alabandina, is a Stone reddifh and blue, as the *Cardius*; and is fo exactly imitated, that, in Colour, the one can fcarcely be diftinguifh'd from the other. It took its Name from a Part of *Afia* fo called, where it was firft found. Its Property is to promote a Flux

of

of Blood. Being drank, it expels and drives out all the Virulence of Poifon I find various Opinions concerning the Colour of this Stone.

Agapis, is a Yellow Stone, of the Colour of a Lion's Skin. It is fo called from *Agape,* which fignifies Love or Charity, becaufe it imports the fame Thing, and Men love it for its Virtue. Being bound to the Wound, it has a wonderful Virtue in curing the Stings of Scorpions and the Bites of Vipers. For being dipp'd in Water, and rubb'd over the Wound, it immediately takes away or mitigates the Pain.

Andromantes, is a Stone of a black Colour, weighty and hard It's faid to attract Silver and Brafs, as the Loadftone does Iron. Being rubbed and put in Water, it emits a bloody Colour like the *Emathites.*

Antracites, or *Antrachas,* is a fparkling Stone of a fiery Colour. It is girdled with a white Vein, cannot bear the Fire, if fmear'd with Oil it lofes its Colour, and if dipp'd in Water, it fparkles the more. *Albertus Magnus* takes it for a *Carbuncle,* but others fay it is not one, tho' it partakes of its Colour and Virtue. Its Virtue is to drive away peftilential Air, and render the Bearer of it fafe It is good in Impoftumes and therefore called

E 3 by

by that Name; in like Manner as we before
spoke of the *Agapis*

Amandinus, is a Stone of a various Colour;
its Virtue is extoll'd for its Efficacy in ex-
pelling Poison, it makes the Wearer of it
victorious, and instructs the Interpreter of
Dreams and Enigmas to solve any Questions
propounded to him about them.

Abeston or *Abestus*, is a Stone of an Iron
Colour, produc'd in *Arcadia* and *Arabia*.
It is called *Abeston*, from its being inex-
tinguishable, for, being set on Fire, it
retains a perpetual Flame. The *Pagans*
made Use of it for Lights in their Temples,
because it preserv'd a most strong and un-
quenchable Flame, not to be extinguish'd
by Showers or Storms It is of a woolly
Texture, and many call it the *Salamander*'s
Feather Its Fire is nourished by an inseparable unctuous Humid flowing from its
Substance; therefore being once kindled it
preserves a constant Light without feeding it
with any Moisture

Asius, is a white Stone and light as the
Pumice, and when lick'd with the Tongue,
has a Salt Taste, being squeez'd in the
Hands, it is easily reduc'd to Dust It is
brought from *Alexandria*; and altho' in
Appearance it is not very promising, yet in

its

its Virtue is very powerful For it cures the Pthifical, being mixed with the Juice of Rofes, in the Manner of an Electuary. It is faid to cure the King's Evil, Fiftulas, the Gout, and many other Diforders; as we find in the Books of Phyficians.

Amianton, is a Stone of a lucid Colour and thready, like feather'd Alumn, but more tenacious Many call it live Flax, for it is only to be wrought upon by being put into the Fire, it emits Threads as from Flax, which proceeds from its infeparable Vifcofity, which fuffers nothing from the Fire, and is fpun like Flax The Antients, when they had a Mind to preferve the Afhes of the Dead, made Sacks of the *Amianton*, and putting the dead Bodies into them, burned them, without hurting the Sack, this they did to prevent any extraneous Matter from mingling with the Afhes of the Deceafed. They fay its Virtue is prevalent againft the Incantations and Sorceries of Magicians.

Augufteum, is a Stone of a black Colour, of the Species of Marbles. It has Spots wavingly difpos'd, in Refemblance of Serpents. It was found in *Egypt* in the Time of *Tiberius Augvftus*, and from him took its Name

Alabafter, or *Alabaftrites*, is a white Stone, circled with white and citron-colour'd Veins.

It

It is of the Marble-kind, and is the beſt for Veſſels to hold Unguents, which are preſerv'd in them without ſpoiling. The beſt Sort is found about *Thebes* and *Damaſcus*, and that which is whiter than the reſt in *India* and *Carmenia*, the baſeſt, without Whiteneſs, in *Cappadocia*. That alſo is the beſt which has the Colour of Honey, with but little Tranſparency *Dioſcorides*, and many other Doctors, account it good in Phyſicks. He who carries it will prove victorious in Suits at Law.

Alabandicus, is a black Stone bordering on the purple, and takes its Name from the Place where it was firſt found. It may be diſſolved by Fire, and poured out like Metal. It is uſeful to Glaſs-makers, to clarify and whiten their Glaſs. It is found in many Places of *Italy*, and is called *Mangadeſus* by the Glaſs-makers.

Aſpilaten, is a Stone in *Arabia*, of a black Colour, generated in the Neſts of *Arabian* Birds, where it is often found. It cures the Splenetick, being bound to the Spleen with the Dung of a Camel.

Abiſtos, is a Stone of a black Colour, ſtreaked with ruddy and ſnowy Veins; being heated in the Fire for eight Days, it retains the Heat in itſelf. It is heavy and

pon-

ponderous, more than the Quantity of it seems to shew.

Asinius, or *Asininus*, a Stone so called from the Ass, because it is taken out of the Woodland or wild Ass. It is whitish, and tending to the Citron, with a round oblongish Figure, of the Bigness of a midling Nut. It is not hard, and has some Crevices which do not penetrate very deep. When broken, it has the Similitude of yellowish lucid Smalt. This Stone is of two Sorts, the Maxillary and Cephalick. The Cephalick being placed on the Head, gives Ease to the Pain of it. The Maxillary cures the Epilepsy, because it is found in the Jaw. It makes the Bearer of it unwearied, so that he shall never faint in Battle, but rather, when his Enemies are tired, he, with recruited Strength, shall smite them with redoubled Fury. Taken with Wine, it drives away Quartan Agues. It is wonderfully efficacious in destroying the Worms in Children. If it be taken in Wine, it corrects the Poison of the Water which has been drank wherein it stood. It is said to assist pregnant Women, and to bring forth the dead Fœtus from the Womb.

Arabica, or *Arabus*, is a Stone of the Colour of Ivory, and takes its Name from *Arabia*, where it is found. It is said to be good

good in nervous Diforders. It is likewife found in *Egypt*. It has the Smell and Colour of Myrrh, and is ufed as a Scent. Being burnt, it is a good Dentifrice.

Amiatus, or *Amianthus*, is a Stone of the Colour of Alumn, it is not to be deftroyed by Fire. It is faid to have Power againft magic Arts; and alfo is extremely ufeful in Medicine

Antiphates, is a Stone of a fhining Black. If it be boil'd in Wine or Milk, it has the Tafte of Myrrh, and is a Defence againft Witchcraft.

Amites, is a Stone of the Colour of Alumn or Nitre, but harder than either. It is generated in *Egypt* or *Arabia*. The *Ethiopic* is green, when diffolved in Water, it takes a milky Colour

Armenus, according to *Aviren*, is a Stone of an azure Colour; tho' others fay it is between a dark Green and a black, and eafily broken; is light in the handling, wants Afperity, and has an admirable Property in curing Melancholy.

Aquilinus, a Lymphatic, is found in a certain Fifh, and is beneficial to the Life of Man. For being hung about the Neck, or otherwife carried, it drives off and takes away the Miferies of a Quartan Ague.

Anancithidus,

Anancithidus, is a Necromantic Stone; whofe Virtue is to call up evil Spirits and Ghofts.

Agirites, is a Stone of the Colour of Silver, with Gold Spots.

Antianeus, is the fame as the *Chrifocolla*.

Aquileus, is the fame as *Ethices*

Androa, is the fame as *Andromadanta*.

B

Balafius, is of a purple or rofy Colour, flames and glitters, and by fome is called the *Placidus*, or *Pleafant* Some think it is the *Carbuncle* diminifh'd in its Colour and Virtue, juft as the Virtue of the Fen ale differs from that of the Male. It is often found that the external Part of one and the fame Stone appears a *Balafius*, and the internal a *Carbuncle*, from whence comes the Saying, that the *Balafius* is the *Carbuncle*'s Houfe The Virtue of the *Balafius* is to overcome and reprefs vain Thoughts and Luxury; to reconcile Quarrels among Friends, and befriends the human Body with a good Habit of Health. Being bruifed and drank with Water, it relieves Infirmities in the Eyes, and gives Help in Diforders of the Liver, and, what is ftill

more

more furprizing, if you touch the four Corners of a Houfe, Garden, or Vineyard, with the *Balafius*, it will preferve them from Lightning, Tempeft and Worms

Beryl, is a Stone of an Olive Colour, or like Sea Water They fay there are nine Species of them, but all of a pale Green. It takes its Name from the Country or Nation where it was found; it has a clear fexagonal Form. *India* produces white *Beryls,* like Sea-water interfected with the Sun-Beams; and fuch are feldom found elfewhere. Curious Antiquity had moft in Efteem thofe that were like the Olive, or the Water of the Sea. But the Moderns value thofe that are of an obfcure chryftal Colour, and fuch by fome are called *Catel* There is another Species which is paler, and called the falfe *Beryl,* which fhines with a Golden or Sky Colour, thefe are from *Babylon*, to which indeed the paler *Chryfopilon* approaches neareft To thefe fucceed the *Hyacinthizontes*, like *Emeralds*; and laftly, the *Heroides* Then the *Cervini*, or tawney Colour, and the dark Olive, and the *Chriftalline* like Chriftal. But the *Indian* are the moft precious of all, as they have a fine Tranfparency, and when they are mov'd the Water feems to move in them, which is

alfo

alſo the Opinion of *Albertus*, tho' he differs from others. But if theſe are roll'd up into the Form of a Ball, and are laid under the Beams of the Sun, they reflect Fire like Concave Mirrors. It has various Virtues. It renders the Bearer of it chearful , preſerves and increaſes Conjugal Love , being hung to the Neck, it drives away idle Dreams , it cures the Diſtempers of the Throat and Jaws, and all Diſorders proceding from the Humidity of the Head, and is a Preſervative againſt them , being taken mixed with an equal Quantity of Silver, it cures the Leproſy. The Water in which it has been put, is good for the Eyes ; and if drank, it diſpels Heavineſs, and cures the Indiſpoſitions of the Liver. It helps pregnant Women in preventing abortive Births, and other Incommodities to which they are liable.

Borax, Noſa, Crapondinus, are ſynonymous Names of the ſame Stone, which is extracted from a Toad : of which there are two Species, the white which is the beſt, and rarely found , the other, is black or dun, with a cerulean Glow, having in the Middle the Similitude of an Eye, and muſt be taken out while the dead Toad is yet panting, and theſe are better than thoſe that are extracted from it after a long Continuance in the Ground.
They

They have a wonderful Efficacy in Poisons. For whoever has taken Poison, let him swallow this , which being down, rolls about the Bowels, and drives out every poisonous Quality that is lodg'd in the Intestines , and then passes thro' the Fundament and is preserv'd. It is an excellent Remedy for the Bites of Reptiles, and takes away Fevers. If it be made into a Lotion and taken, it is a great Help in Disorders of the Stomach and Reins ; and some say, it has the same Effect if carried about one.

Bezoar, is a red, dusty, light, and brittle Stone ; by some it is described as of a Citron Colour. All agree that it obtains the first Place in Remedies against Poisons. For a Dram of it taken, entirely expels the Poison whatever it be. And hence, for its Excellence, every Thing that frees the Body from any Ailment, is called the *Bezoar* of that Ailment. And thus its Name is become general, as is held by the *Conciliator* concerning Poisons, and by many other learned Men

Bolus Armenus, is a Vein of Earth found in *Armenia*, and altho' it is not a Stone, yet for its noble Virtue, is numbred among Stones The Colour of it is reddish inclining to a Citron with a green Dusk. Its Complexion

plexion is cold and dry. It is an excellent Remedy in Pestilential Fevers and Fluxes of the Belly. It helps Emoptoics, the Splenetick, and such as are disorder'd in the Stomach. It is very much adulterated, and there is scarce any true and genuine to be had, nor did I ever see any good.

Beloculus, is a white Stone, having a black Pupil. For its Beauty the *Syrians* put it in the Ornaments of the Sacrifices to the God *Belus* It is said to render the Bearer of it invisible in a Field Battle

Basanites, or *Basaltem,* is a Stone of an iron Colour, is found in *Egypt* and *Ethiopia,* and when bruised in Water emits a Saffron Colour.

Bronia, has the Likeness of the Head of a Shell, its Virtue is, to resist Lightnings.

Batanites, is a Stone of two Species, the one is green, the other has the Colour of Brass, with a flaming Vein running thro' the Middle of it.

C

Carbuncle, and by some called *Anthrax,* brandishes its fiery Rays, of a Violet Colour, on every Side; and in the Dark appears
like

like a fiery Coal. It is efteemed the firft
among burning Gems, both for Colour,
Beauty, and Price. There are Twelve
Species of it. The nobler Sort are found
in *Libia* among the *Troglodites*. It is not
hurt by Fire, nor does it take the Colour
of another Gem that is put to it, tho' other
Gems receive from it. It is alfo Male and
Female; in the Males, the Stars appear
burning within them, but the Females throw
out their Brightnefs, and fome fay that
thofe of *India*, are more valuable than the
reft. Altho' we have faid that there are
twelve Species of the fiery Sort, yet we fhall
take Notice only of five of the moft remarkable of them. The *Carbuncle* obtains the
firft Place, the *Ruby* follows; the *Balafius* is
likewife reckon'd of this Species, the *Rubith*
is the fame as the *Spinella*, and has the
fourth Place, and the *Granate* is number'd
among the laft. The virtual Power of the
Carbuncle is to drive away poifonous and
infectious Air, to reprefs Luxury, to give
and preferve the Health of the Body. It
takes away vain Thoughts, reconciles Differences among Friends, and makes a mighty
Increafe of Profperity

    Calcedonius, or *Calcedon*, as fome call it,
is of a pale Colour, but the Saphirine is the
beft;

beſt ; the Learned reckon three Species of
ſpecial Note, tho' ſome ſay there are more ,
for at this Time, Germany produces ſuch a
Diverſity of Species, that it would be in
vain to enumerate them. The Saphirine
obtains the firſt Place , the pale duſky,
bordering on the white, follows , the laſt is
a dead red, not tranſparent Very often
theſe Species are mixed, and the different
Colours are found in one and the ſame
Stone ; but Ethiopia produces the moſt
perfect of all Are there not likewiſe found
on the Shore of the Adriatic Sea, near your
City, the Calcedonian pale white, and alſo
the hardeſt dun ? Being hung about the
Neck, they drive away fantaſtical Illuſions
occaſion'd by Melancholy. If a Perſon
carries about him one of them perforated,
with the Hairs of an Aſs run thro', he will
be ſuccefsful in Civil Cauſes and Contentions.
It preſerves the Strength of the Body The
black or Saphirine prevent hoarſeneſs and
clear the Voice All the Species of it bridle
Luſt , and is a Preſervative from Tempeſts
and ſiniſter Events.

Chelidonius, is a Stone found in the Stomach
of a young Swallow , and is of two Species.
That which is red, if carried in a clean
Linen Cloth, is of Service to mad People

I   and

and Lunaticks, and eradicates periodical Diforders It renders thofe who wear it eloquent
and acceptable.   Being bruifed to Pieces in
Water, and made into a Pellet, it cures the
Diftempers of the Eyes.   But the black con-
ducts Affairs undertaken to a happy Iffue.
It quells Anger, and makes the Bearer of it
agreeable and pleafant, and appeafes the
Wrath of Mafters.   Being tied about the
Neck in a yellow Linen Cloth, it drives a-
way Fevers, and puts a Stop to and brings
down all noxious Humours.   It has been experienced, that if it be hung about the
Neck, it cures the Epilepfy, or Falling-
Sicknefs, and the Jaundice.   Some fay, it
fhould be wrapt in the Skin of a Calf, or a
flung Hart, and bound to the left Arm Such
Stones ought to be extracted while the young
Brood ftand in their Neft, and if taken in
the Month of *Auguft*, they will be the more
perfect, provided the young Birds do not
touch the Earth, nor their Dams be prefent
when they are extracted

Coral grows in the Sea like a Tree, but
without Leaves, in Magnitude not exceeding
two Feet   Of this there are two Species, the
Red and White, tho' *Avicen* holds there is
a third Species, which is Black   I once faw
the White and Red join'd on one Stem.

The

The White indeed are often perforated, and are good for nothing; but thofe which are perfectly white, and the reddeft, are the beft. Their Virtues, but chiefly of the Red, is to ftop every Flux of Blood. Being carried about one, or wherever it be in a Houfe or Ship, it drives away Ghofts, Hobgoblins, Illufions, Dreams, Lightnings, Winds and Tempefts *Metbrodorus* calls it the *Gorgon*, which he interprets of its refifting Whirlwinds and Lightnings, and that it protects from every Incurfion of wild Beafts It gives Relief in Pains of the Stomach and Heart. Being hung down upon the Stomach, or taken internally, it helps the Weaknefs thereof. It is good for an Impoftume in the Spleen or Inteftines It makes found the wafted Gums, cleanfes putrid Sores, and repreffes any hurtful Medicine. The Shavings or Scrapings of it, drank with Wine, are good againft the Gravel Being broke to pieces and ftrewn, or hung up among Fruit-bearing Trees, or difperfed with Seed in a Field, it gives Fertility, and keeps off Hail and blighting Winds I have had it from a creditable Perfon, and have often experienced it myfelf, that it will prevent Infants, juft born, from falling into an Epilepfy Let there be put in the Mouth of the Child, before it has tafted

F 2   any

any Thing, half a Scruple of the Powder of Red Coral, and let it be fwallowed; for it is a wonderful Preferver. Many of its Virtues I omit for the Sake of Brevity.

Cornelian, is a Stone of a reddifh or ruddy Colour, and fuch are Orientals, they which are found in the River *Rhine*, are perfectly red, having as it were the Colour of Vermillion Some border upon a clear Citron, fome are like the Wafhing of Flefh It reftrains menftruous Fluxes, and ftops the Hemorrhoids. It cures the Bloody Flux; and being worn about the Neck, or on the Finger, it affwages Strife and Anger.

Cryftal, is a Stone like Ice, both in Colour and Tranfparency, with a pretty good Hardnefs Some imagine it is Snow turn'd to Ice, and been hardening for thirty Years, and turn'd to a Rock by Age. Others fay, it acquires its Lapidity from Earthinefs and not from Coldnefs Some, on the contrary, affirm, that thefe, like other Stones, are generated with much Water, for this Reafon, That the Cryftal is never found in the Meridional Parts where there is no Snow They are the more confirm'd in this Opinion, when they fee it in the Northern *Alps* where the Snow and Ice are perpetual, where the Sun, in the hotteft Seafon, darts his moft fervent Rays

Rays but very obliquely from the Elevation of
the Pole; and there abounds the greatest
Quantity of Cryftal. It is geneiated likewife in *Afia* and *Cyprus*, but the moft excellent are produc'd on the Tops of the *Alps*,
in *Ethiopia*, and in an Ifland of the Red
Sea, called *Meron*, fituated on the Frontier
of *Arabia*. *Scythia* likewife abounds with
Cryftal, us'd for the making of Cups
A Ball made out of Cryftal, and expos'd to
the Sun, inflames any combuftible Matter
that is put under it, but not before the Ball
is heated. This is eafily accounted for by
Philofophers, but is not the Subject of our
prefent Enquiry. Cryftal being hung about
thofe that are afleep, keeps off bad Dreams;
diffolves Spells; being held in the Mouth,
it affuages Thirft, and when bruifed with
Honey, fills the Breafts with Milk But
the principal Ufe of Cryftal is for making
of Cups, rather than any Thing elfe it is
good for.

Crifopraffus, or *Crifopreffus*, is a Stone of a
green Colour, like the Juice of Cyprefs,
with golden Drops appearing in it, from
whence it takes its Name. For *Crifos*, in
Greek, fignifies Gold, and this Stone is compofed of a gold and green Colour *India*
and *Ethiopia* produce it Its principal Virtue

F 3   is

is to cherish the Sight. It gives Assiduity
in good Works, it banishes Covetousness;
makes the Heart glad, and removes Uneasi-
nesses from it

Crisoletus, *Crisolenus* or *Crisoensis*, is a
transparent Stone, sparkling with Gold and
Fire. But it's properly called *Chrisoletus*,
taking its Name from the *Greek Crisos*, in
the *Latin*, signifying Gold, and *oletus* whole;
hence *Crisoletus*, or wholly Gold. The
Ethiopic are the best. The *Indian* and *Arabic*
are not quite so lucid and transparent, having
in them a dusky Cloud and likewise border
upon the Citron. The *Ethiopic*, in a Morning, seem as if they were on Fire, but in the
Day they appear like Gold. A *Crisolete*
bound round with Gold, and carried in the
left Hand, drives away Night-hags, and
dispels Fears and melancholy Illusions. It
is particularly efficacious in rendering in-
effectual the Incantations and Enchantments
of those detestable Creatures call'd Witches.
It being bor'd thro', and the Hairs of an
Ass pass'd thro' it, its Virtue is the greater
in driving away evil Spirits. If held in the
Hand, it extinguishes a feverish Heat

Crisolitus, of this Stone there is one Kind,
of a gold Colour, with some burning Sparks
But there is another, which indeed is the

most

moſt generally eſteem'd, which is azure and green, like the Water of the Sea in its greateſt Greenneſs. Being placed under the Rays of the Sun, it repreſents a Golden Star. It is found in *Ethiopia*. Being ſet in Gold it prevails againſt nocturnal Terrors. It gives Wiſdom and Honour, and turns away Folly. Being bruiſed and drank, it helps the Aſthmatic.

Celonites, or *Celontes*, is, as ſome will have it, of three Kinds. It is extracted from a large Tortoiſe, and has a Shell of a Pearl Colour. This Sort is ſpotted and purple, and its Property is to ſit. The Virtue of it deſerves particular Regard, for whoever ſhall at a proper Time, having firſt waſh'd his Mouth, carry it under his Tongue, will preſently feel in himſelf a kind of divine Inſpiration to foretel future Events. Such Times are theſe. The whole Day of the firſt of the New Moon, and for the fifteen Days following during the Lunar Aſcenſion, every Day from Sun riſing till Six o'Clock. But in the Decreaſe, it pours forth the Effect of its Virtue all the Time before Day. The other two Stones are Cephalic and Hepatic, whoſe Virtues are not trivial. The Cephalic, is ſo called from the Place where it is found, *i. e.* the Head, and is good for the Head ach,

F 4
and

and refifts Lightnings. The Hepatic is likewife fo call'd from the Place where it is found, *i e* the Liver Being bruifed and drank with Water juft before the Coming on of a Quartan Ague, it wonderfully prevents it. Thefe Stones are likewife called *Drome.* Being carried with a Root of Piony, it makes thofe who carry them Mafters of their Defires.

Cogolites, or *Cegolites,* is, by Phyficians, reckon'd a *Jewifh* Stone, from its being frequently found in that Country, and like the Nut of an Olive, but in the Infide it has the Colour of Alumn or Silver It is not grateful to the Sight, but is ufeful in Medicine. Being bruifed and diffolv'd in Water, and taken inwardly, it diffolves Stones in the Kidneys, and clears the Bladder from Gravel, and being drank with a proper Quantity of Water, removes the Strangury

Ceraunius, or *Cerraclus,* is a Stone of a pyramidal Form There are two Kinds of them, the one is cryftalline tinged with Saffron, the other of the Colour of the *Pyrites.* They are faid to fall from the Clouds, and in a Place neat where has been a Stroke of Thunder. The *German* is the Prime, the *Spanifh* is the Second, which flafhes like a Flame of Fire *Socatus* tells us of another Species, which is black. *Evax*

con-

contradicts thefe, when he fays they are of divers Colours, but the hardeft has a great Virtue. For it preferves the Bearer of it from Drowning, and from being hurt by a Whirlwind or Lightning; it gives fweet and pleafant Dreams

Corvina, is a Stone found in the Head of the Fifh *Cabot*, and are always two. The Colour of it is a darkifh white, with an oblong crooked Figure in one part, and in the other concave, with a little rifing in the Middle. It is extracted while the Fifh is yet panting, in the Increafe of the Moon, and in the Month of *May* Being carried in fuch a Manner as it may touch the Flefh, it cures the Gripes; and being bruifed and taken, it has the fame Effect.

Cimedia, is taken out of the Brain of a Fifh of the fame Name, there are two found in the Head, and a third near the third Joint of the Backbone, towards the Tail; it is round, and of the Length of feven Fingers Its broad Head being put before the Light, the Spine appears within. Magicians fay, that their Virtue is to foretel the Calms and Storms of the Sea and Air. If taken in Drink they excite Luxury in the Day.

Cal-

Calchophanus, is black ; and being carried in the Mouth, preferves the Windpipe from Hoarfenefs, and makes the Voice fonorous.

Caldaicus, or *Callayca,* is of a green Pale and dull, not limpid, nor pleafant to the Sight, but is a Stone that looks well in Gold ; and in the cold Rocks in *Media* and *Germany,* it fhoots out itfelf like an Eye.

Crifocollus, is a Stone of the Likenefs of Gold The Province of *Media* produces it, where the Pifmires throw up the Gold. It has the Virtue of the Magnet, and increafes Gold.

Crifoprafius, is a Stone which fhines in the dark, of an ebbing and confufed Colour, like rotten Oak put in an obfcure Place ; but in the Light, it is faint, of the Colour of pale Gold, without any Brightnefs.

Chemites, is a Stone that has the Refemblance of Ivory, not heavy, and in Hardnefs like Marble. It is faid to preferve the Bodies of the Dead a long Time from being hurt by the Worms, and from Putrefaction

Crifonterinus, borders upon a gold Colour, and is brittle. Tho' it be an unpolifh'd Stone, yet it has no contemptible Virtue. Being hung about the Neck, it cures the Pthifical, and, after the fame Manner, it

removes

removes the Pain which Children feel in breeding Teeth.

Cysteolithos, has a Mixture of Whiteness with the Citron, and is found in a Sea Sponge, and tho' it be somewhat unsightly, it helps those troubled with the Stone, if drank in strong Wine, and if hung about the Necks of Children, it takes away the Cough

Catochites, by some is taken, tho' falsly, for the *Sagda* According to *Solinus,* it is to be found in *Corsica,* it separates any glutinous Thing that sticks to the Hands of him that touches it, and then fastens itself to the Body like Glew It makes a Man victorious in Contests, and by taking one Scruple of it, it is powerful against magic Arts

Corvia, or *Corvina,* is a Stone of a reddish Colour, and accounted artificial On the Calends of *April,* boil the Eggs taken out of a Crow's Nest, till they are hard; and being cold, let them be placed in the Nest as they were before When the Crow knows this, she flies a long Way to find this Stone, and having found it, returns to the Nest, and the Eggs being touch'd with it, they become fresh and prolifick. The Stone must immediately be snatch'd out of the Nest.

Its

Its Virtue is to increase Riches, to beſtow Honours, and to foretel many future Events.

Cambnites, is a Stone of a cryſtal Colour ſomewhat obſcure. He who carries it, will pleaſe Men, and be affable and amiable to all. If bound to the left Arm, it cures the Dropſical I believe indeed it is the ſame as the *Kebrates*

Cepocapites, or *Cepites*, is a white Stone, having Knots with Veins of white Marble. A Group of Images of divers Things is figur'd in it, as in the *Achates*

Calorites, is of a green Colour, like Juice preſs'd from the Herb. Magicians report, that it is taken out of the Belly of the Bird *Silta* If bound with Iron, it is powerful in magic Arts.

Cepenalus, is a Stone of many Colours, and tranſparent, reflecting the Similitude of the Beholder, ſometimes in the Manner of a Jaſper, then as a Cryſtal, and ſometimes as a Diamond

Corintheus, is of the Marble Kind, and of a citron Colour, diverſify'd into other Colours. It takes its Name from *Corinth*, where there is found great Plenty of it It is fit for Buildings, and Pillars, Threſholds, Beams, and many other Things have, for a long Courſe of Time, been made of it.

Cy-

Cyanica, or *Cyaneus*, is an azure Stone, glittering with purple Beams, vary'd with golden Stars, and sometimes appears with little shining Points intermixed of divers Colours It is found in *Scythia*, and is Male and Female. The Male is neater and purer than the Female, and is beautified with the Intermixture of small golden Dust

Caristeus, is of a green Colour, taking its Name from its Aspect, because it is grateful to the Sight, which it comforts with its Greenness.

Calaminaris, is a Stone, yellow, tender, not lucid, nor transparent. If it be drenched nine Times in Vinegar, and finely pulveriz'd with the Blood of a Fowl, it makes a fine Eye Salve

Crisopassus, according to *Solinus*, is a Species of *Beryl*, having a gold Colour mixed with purple.

Coaspis, is of a green Colour, with the Brightness of Gold, and took its Name from a River of the *Persians*, where it was found.

Cimilianitus, is of the Colour of Marble, having in the Middle a golden Pupil, or of a Saffron Colour, and is found in the Channel of the River *Euphrates*.

Crisolansis is the same as *Crisoletus*.

Crisites, is a Stone of the Colour of an

Oyster,

Oyſter, and is found in *Egypt.*

Criſopilon, is a Species of *Beryl,* as hath been before ſhewn under that Head.

Criſoberillus; ſee before under the Head of *Beryl*

Coranus, is white, of the Marble Kind, and harder than Parian

Criſopis, is a Stone that looks like Gold.

Carcina, is a Stone of the Colour of a Crab

Crapondinus, is the ſame as *Borax*

Cilicolus, is the ſame as *Beloculus*

Chryſotopteron, is a Species of the *Topaz,* and like *Criſopraſſius*

D

Demonius is a Stone mixed with a double Colour like the Rainbow, from which it took its Name, for that is called the Demoniacal Bow It is ſaid to be a powerful Relief againſt Agues, expels Poiſon, and renders the Bearer of it ſafe from, and a Conqueror over his Enemies

Dionyſia, is black, with red Spots ſcatter'd over it Some ſay, it has a brown or iron Colour, ſprinkled over with ſnow Spots. It is found in the Eaſt, and if it be diſſolved in Water, it gets the Smell of Wine; and

with

with its Odor difperfes Drunkennefs, and overcomes, and caufes the Odor of the Wine to evaporate

Diacodas, or *Diacodus,* is like *Beryl* in Colour, with a Palenefs It difturbs Devils beyond all others, as in fome Meafure may be made appear For if it be thrown in Water, with the Words of its Charm fung, it fhews various Images of Devils, and gives Anfwers to thofe that queſtion it Being held in the Mouth , a Man may call any Devil out of Hell, and receive Satisfaction to fuch Que-ſtions as he may aſk. It abhors the Bodies of the Dead , for if you fhould touch the Body of a dead Perfon with it, you will foon deprive it of its Virtue

Draconites, or *Dentrites,* or *Draeonius,* or *Obfianus,* and is alfo called the *Evening Ki-medius,* is a Stone lucid and tranfparent, of a criftalline Colour. *Albertus Magnus* fays, it is of a black Colour, and that its Figure is pyramidal, and not lucid. Some fay, it fhines like a Looking glafs, with a Blacknefs ; which many feek after, but never find. It is brought from the Faſt, where there are great Dragons, for s aken out of the Head of Dragons or I wale the Beaſt is yet parting les its Virtue if it remains in the Head any Time after the

Death

Death of the Dragon. Some bold Fellows, in thofe Eaftern Parts, fearch out the Dens of the Dragons, and in thefe they ftrew Grafs, mixed with foporiferous Medicaments ; which the Dragons, when they return to their Dens, eat and are thrown into a Sleep, and in that Condition they cut off their Heads, and extract the Stone It has a rare Virtue in fubduing all Sorts of Poifon, efpecially that of Serpents It alfo renders the Poffeffor of it bold and invincible, for which Reafon, the Kings of the Eaft boaft they have fuch a Stone.

Drofolitus, is a Stone of a various Colour, and derives its Name from itfelf, for if it be put near the Fire, it emits a Kind of Sweat.

Doriatides, is a Stone found in the Head of a Cat, fuddenly cut off, and given to the Pifmires to eat, and the Colour of it is black and fhining Some will have it to be extracted from the Head of a Cock, as hereafter, under the Head *Radain* Its Virtue is to perfect all our Wifhes, and obtain all our Defires

Doctus, is a green Stone, fomewhat clear, and I am apt to think is the *Crifolitus*, as before mentioned

Ethiopia,

E.

Elitropia, or *Elitropus,* is a green Gem,
and, as fome fancy, like an Emerald, fprinkled with bloody Spots. But Necromancers
call it the *Babylonian* Gem, and is found
in *Africa* and *Ethiopia* The Caufe of its
Name is taken from its Effeſt. This is
the readieſt Way of knowing it. If it be put
into Water in a Bafon, which has been
firſt rubbed over with the Juice of the
Herb of its own Name, and fet undei the
Rays of the Sun, the Water will appear ied,
and the Sun bloody, as if it fuffeied an Eclipfe.
At length the Water will bubble up, and
run over the Bafon, as if it had been work'd
up by Fire Being placed out of the Water,
it receives the Sun in the Manner of a Mirror.
So that by infpeſting the *Elitropia,* we may
fee the Solar Eclipfes. It is likewife found
in *Cyprus,* but the nobler Sort, as *Solinus*
teftifies, is in *Lybia.* Magicians report, that
if it be confecrated with a certain Verfe, and
infcribed with certain Chaiaſters, it will
enable the Owner of it to foretel future
Things ; and if it be iubb'd over with the
Juice of the Herb of its own Name, it de-
ceives the Sight, in fuch a Manner, as that

G   it

it renders the Bearer of it invifible. The Virtue of it is, to procure Safety and long Life to the Poffeffor of it ; and likewife ftops any Flux of Blood. Poifons alfo fubmit to it.

Emathitis, or *Emathites*, is a reddifh Stone, obfcure and hard, having the Brightnefs of Iron, with Veins of Blood, and ftains the Hands of him that touches it with a bloody Colour. It claims its Name from its Virtue. For *Emeth* fignifies Blood, and *Titel* ftopping, for its principal Virtue is to ftop Bleeding. There are five Species of it, and called after the Names of the Countries where they are found. The *Arabic* and *African* are preferable to all the reft. The *Phrygian* and *Ethiopic* are of meaner Account, although *Socatus* may be of a contrary Opinion. The *German* is the bafeft of all. Its Virtue is Stiptic, if it be wafhed according to medicinal Art. But *Galen* holds, that it is warming and extenuating, which muft not be underftood of that which is wafhed. It is a moft excellent Remedy for the Emoptoics, fuch as are troubled with the Bloody Flux, and the Menfes, if it be ground in a Mortar with a proper Liquor till it acquires a bloody Colour. If to what has been before-mention'd be added, the white of an Egg, or Honey, or the Juice of a red Apple, it heals the
fharp

ſharp Humour of the Eyes and Darkneſs of the Sight. Being drank with Wine, it helps thoſe that are wounded with the Stings of Serpents. The Duſt of it likewiſe cures fungous Fleſh If mixed with Honey, it is uſeful for thoſe that are troubled with bad Eyes. It is alſo ſaid to diſſolve the Stone in the Bladder, and if put over hot Water, it grows warm, and throws out a Heat. The *Phrygian* is burnt, to make it the more efficacious for the Purpoſes aforeſaid.

Ethices, or *Endes*, by ſome called *Aquileus*, is a Stone of a Scarlet Colour It is called *Aquileus*, becauſe ſometimes the Eagles on the Shore of the *Perſian* Ocean, put it in their Neſts among their Eggs. It is likewiſe called *Pragnus*, becauſe it contains a little Stone within it, as if it were pregnant, and is heard to rattle, and, as I ſaid, ſome deſcribe it of a Scarlet Colour; others indeed ſay it is more like Fleſh, plain, lucid, and of a moderate Bigneſs Some ſay it has an oblong Figure, inclining to Roundneſs This Variety of Opinions in Authors ariſes from the Variety of Places where it is found. Its Virtue is admirable. For ſome ſay, if it be held out to one that has poiſon'd Meat in his Hand, he will not be able to ſwallow it ; the Stone being removed, he may take

it. Some fay, it muft be put into the Meat.
Being tied to the left Arm of a pregnant
Woman, it prevents Abortion. And if in
the Hour of Birth, it be bound to the Thigh,
it removes Dangers, and accelerates the Birth.
It helps thofe who are troubled with the Epilepfy. It drives away poifonous Creatures ;
and therefore Eagles lay it in their Nefts, that
their Eggs and Young may be preferved untouch'd by venemous Animals. It makes
the Bearer of it amiable, fober, and rich,
and preferves him from adverfe Cafualties.

Enydros, or *Eryndros*, is a Stone of a
chriftal Colour, and has its Name from the
Greek Word, *Hydros*, which fignifies Water,
and is perpetually diftilling Drops : The
Caufe of which is not urknown to Philofophers ; for as it is of an exceeding cold Nature, it does, with its Frigidity, convert the
Air, which continually touches it, into
Water. It is good in burning Fevers

Epiftides, or *Epiftrites*, is in its Colour
red and glittering. It has its Birth in *Corinth*.
They fay, if it be faften'd over the Heart with
magical Bands, and repeating proper Verfes,
it will keep a Man fafe from every Misfor-
tune. It drives away Locufts and mifchie-
vous Birds, blighting Winds, and Storms.

Ex-

Exacolitus, is a Stone of many and various Colours mingled one with another It has a folutive Virtue, as fkilful Phyficians fay, and being diffolved in Wine and drank, it helps thofe that are troubled with the Cholic and Iliac Paffion.

Eftimion, or *Exmiffon*, is of a moft agreeable Afpect, glittering with a gold and fiery Colour, and carries a white Light in its Extremity.

Execonthalitus, or *Hexaconta*, is a Stone having in the Compafs of a little Orb, fixty diftinct Colours. It is frequently found in *Lybia*. So many Virtues are afcribed to it, as demonftrate it to contain the Ornaments of precious Stones.

Exebonos, or *Exebenus*, is white and fair; with which Goldfmiths ufe to burnifh their Gold. Being bruifed and drank, it cures thofe that are mad It heals Pains in the Stomach, and cherifhes the Fœtus in the Womb. It diffolves the Stone in the Bladder, if bound to the Thigh, it haftens the Birth ; and reftrains Lechery.

Eumetis, is of the Colour of Flint. Being put under the Head of one who is fleeping, it makes nocturnal Dreams like Oracles.

Emites, has the Colour of Ivory, and is like white Marble, but of a lefs Hardnefs.

It

It is said, that the Sepulcher of King *Darius* was made of it.

Egyptilla, is a black Stone, having an azure Superficies, with gold Veins; and takes its Name from the Place where it is found. If bruised in Water, it yields a Saffron Colour and the Taste of Wine.

Emerrem, is a Gem of a grassy Colour, which the *Assyrians* say, is sacred to God; it is a superstitious Gem.

Effestis, or *Effestites*, is a Stone that has the Nature of a Mirror, and reflects Images, and is found in *Corinth*. They say, if it be put in hot Water, it grows warm, and being opposed to the Sun, kindles Fire in Matter put in a Disposition for it.

Elopsites, is a Stone with no Ornament, but supplies in Virtue what is deficient in Beauty. Being hung about the Head, it cures the Head ach.

Eunophius, is like the *Ethices*, as it sounds inwardly. Some think it is the same, and of like Efficacy.

Electioni, is the same as the *Gagates*.

Echistes, the same as *Ethices*.

Echidnes, is a Stone with Serpentine Spots.

Fila-

F

Filaterius, is a Stone of the Colour of the *Crifolite* ; it difperfes Terrors and melancholic Paffions , gives Chearfulnefs and Wifdom ; renders the Bearer thereof complaifant, and comforts the Spirits

Fingites, is of a white Colour, hard as Marble, and tranfparent like Alabafter; it is brought from *Cappadocia* Some report, that a certain King built a Temple of this Stone, without Windows , and from its Tranf-parency, the Day was admitted into it in fo clear a Manner as if it had been all open.

Fongites, is a Stone of whofe Colour there is no fmall Doubt among the Learned. I think this may proceed from the Diverfity of its Species. Some fay, it is like burning Gems; others that it is of a chriftalline Colour, and in the Infide, like Flame. It is found in *Perfia*. Its Virtue is not affigned by many. But *Evax* tells us, that if any one carries a red *Fongites* in his Hand, it removes the Ailments of the Body, and affuages Anger

Falcones, or *Urpine*, vulgarly *Arfenick* , if it be whiten'd by Sublimation, it inclines to a golden red Colour, and takes the Nature

G 4   of

of Sulphur, and by Alchymifts is called one of the Spirits   It has a warming and drying Virtue, and by Calcination acquires Blacknefs; but after Sublimation it has a Whitenefs; and when it is fublimated three or four Times, it becomes aduft in the higheft Degree; fo that it corrodes all Metals except Gold. Being pulveriz'd, and put into a Wound, it eats away the proud Flefh.   Taken inwardly, it is Poifon to all Animals.

Frigius, is a green Stone, and being burnt acquires a Rednefs   It is good for painting Cloth; and much ufed in Medicine, as *Diofcorides* faith; for it cures Fiftulas and the Gout.

G

Granate, is reckon'd among the burning Gems, and a Stone of the Carbuncle Kind; there are three Species of it.   A dark Red like the Flower of a Pomegranate Apple. Another is of a red Colour, and a little bordering on the Citron, fomewhat like a *Jacinth*. The third Species, which is called *Surian*, is of a reddifh Violet, and this is efteem'd more precious than the reft, and is found in *Ethiopia*, among the Sands of the Sea   Its Virtue is to chear the Heart and drive away Sorrow.

Sorrow. Some fay, it defends the Bearer of it from peftilential Difeafes

Galactides, or *Galaricides*, is a Stone of an Afh Colour, or, as fome fancy, white milky Colour, it is found in the *Nile* and in the River *Athaleus*. If it be bruifed in Water, it gives the Colour and Tafte of Milk There are fome who call this an *Emerald* compafs'd about with white Veins. It is differently named from the Diverfity of its Virtue. Some call it *Elebron*, Magicians *Senochites*, others *Graffites*, fome *Galbates* or *Anachites*. Magicians infinitely extol this Stone, for it makes magical Writings to be heard, and Ghofts call'd up to return Anfwers. It alfo buries in Oblivion Quarrels and Mifchiefs formerly done. He who carries it about him, and fhould happen to offend the King or any other Perfon, it will prefently pacify and bring him to a benevolent Temper. It makes a Man victorious in Caufes, witty, amiable and eloquent, and is a Protection againft Witchcraft. Being hung about the Neck, it fills the Breafts with Milk. If tyed to the Thigh with a woollen Thread, it facilitates the Birth of a pregnant Ewe; but if held in the Mouth till it melts, it difturbs the Mind If bruifed and mixed with Salt, and ftiewed

over

over a foul Sheepfold, as the *Egyptian* Shepherds say, it fills the Udders of the Sheep with Milk and makes them fruitful, and frees them from the Mange. They say likewise, that it cures the Itch in Man. Being bound to a Tooth, it takes away its stinking Smell If three Times bruised with Water and dried, and given to drink in clear Water, it heals Discords. It joins in Love two who are at Variance, so that their Love will afterwards be inseparable.

Garatronicus, or, as some, *Galgatromeus*, is a reddish Stone, sprinkled with small Saffron Veins, and like the Skin of a Kid. This is useful for military Men. It is reported that *Achilles* had it, and carried it with him to the War, that he was never foil'd by any Man, but always came off victorious; but happening to be without it he fell by his Enemies. The Easterns have great Quantities of them, and make Hilts for their Swords of it, that so they may never be without it when they go into Battle, since its Virtue is to render the Bearer of it Conqueror.

Galatides, or *Galactica*, or *Gelatia*, and many other Names it is called by, is a white lucid Stone, in Form of an Acorn, hard as the Adamant, and so cold that it can

hardly

hardly be warmed by Fire; which proceeds from the exceeding Clofenefs of its Pores, which will not fuffer the Heat of the Fire to penetrate Its Coldnefs bridles Luxury and reftrains Anger, and yields a Remedy for all the feverifh Indifpofitions of the human Body.

Gelachides, or *Garatides*, is a Stone of a dark Colour, and renders the Bearer of it amiable, mild and gracious Being held in the Mouth, it makes a Man give true Judgment, and rightly diftinguifh between various Opinions, and will let him know what another thinks of him. The Learned fay, we may know fuch a Stone by Trial Thus, if a human Body be fmeared with Honey, and put in a Place where there are Flies, if this Stone be held in the Hand, and it is a genuine *Garatides*, the Body remains untouch'd by the Flies and Bees, and when the Stone is let go, it will be molefted

Gargates, tho' by many it is accounted a Gum, yet it is numbred among Stones, and takes its Name from the Place where it is found. There are two Species of it; the Citron, which is called Amber, of which we fhall fpeak hereafter, the other is black, and by many called black Amber, and this is properly the *Gargates*, tho' *Pliny* greatly differs from others, it is found in *Lycia*.

Solinus

Solinus affirms, it is found in *Britain* in great Plenty. The *Gargates*, as I said, is black, light, dry, and lucid, not transparent, and if put into Fire, has, as it were, the Smell of Pitch. Being heated with rubbing, it attracts Straws and Chaff. The Smoak of it drives away Devils, and dissolves Spells and Enchantments, and helps the Dropsical. Being bruised in Water, and given to a pregnant Woman, it brings forward the Fœtus; and in whatever Manner it is drank by a Woman, it makes her void foul Urine; but has no such Effect on a Virgin. If used as a Perfume, it is said to provoke the Menses in Women, to cure the Epilepsy, to drive away Serpents, and to heal their Bite if mixed with the Marrow of a Stag, and fastens loose Teeth.

Gerades, is a red glittering Stone, and if oppos'd to the Sun, darts out fiery Rays. Its Virtue is to defend a Man from Birds of Prey.

Gallerica, is a green Stone, pale and too thick, not pleasant, bedeck'd with Gold, from whence it is named

Garamantica, is like the Emerald, and has a cross white Line; it is of great Use in the magic Art.

Gasidana, is a Stone of a Swan Colour.
This

This Gem is likewife faid to conceive, and being fhook, confeffes it has a Birth within it, fome think it is the *Ethices*.

Grogius, is the fame as *Coral*; it takes its Name from its Power of ftopping Thunder and Lightning

Glofopetra, or *Gulofus*, is a Stone like the human Tongue, from whence it took its Name. They fay, it is not bred in the Earth, but in the Wane of the Moon falls from Heaven. Magicians attribute to it an extraordinary Efficacy in their Art, for by it they fay, the Lunar Motions are excited.

Grifoletus, is the fame as the *Crifolete*.

Garamantides, the fame as *Sandaftros*.

Galaxia, is a black Stone, with bloody and white Veins interwoven in it.

Galacidem, is the fame as the Emerald.

H

Hyena, is a precious Stone and worthy to be preferved. It is denominated from the Beaft of its own Name, in whofe Eyes it is found. It is of many Colours The Ufe of it, if Report be true, is, That if the Mouth be wafhed, and it is put under the Tongue, it will immediately make the Perfon foretel future Things. Whoever carries it about

him

him will never have the Quartan Ague, nor
the Gout

Hieracites, is varied in its Colour, like
the Wing of a Hawk. Some say, it is of a
black Colour, and that it is the same as the
Gelachides, since it has the same Virtue

Hamonis, is a Stone of a gold Colour, and
is numbred among the moſt sacred Gems
It has the Shape of a Ram's Horn, and is
found in *Ethiopia* If a Man puts himself in
a Poſture of Contemplation, it gives the
Mind a Repreſentation of all divine Things

Hormesion, is a Stone of the moſt agreeable Aſpect, glittering with a fiery and golden
Colour, and emitting a white Light

Horcus, is a Stone which the *Alexandrians*
call *Catimia* ; it is black, and eaſily broken.
It enters into the ſolid Parts of Silver

Hyſmeri, is the same as the *Smeriglius*.

Hammochryſos, is a Stone having ſquare
golden Sands mixed in its Subſtance.

I

Jacinth, to which Antiquity has aſſigned
three Species, which take their Names from
their ſhining Quality For ſome of them are
of a Citron Colour, others of a Granate,
others blue, and all tranſparent, and are
well

well enough known from their Denomination.
For the Citron are of a citron Colour; the
Granate, of the Colour of the Flower of a
Pomegranate Apple, and the Blue of an
azure Colour, which in the Mouth feel
colder than the others, and thefe are likewife called aquatic To thefe fome add
another Species, which they call the Saphirine. All of them, however, have a Rednefs and Yellownefs mixed with the aforefaid
Colours. This Stone above all others, delights in Day light, but fades in Darknefs.
Thofe are reckon'd the beft, whofe Colour
is neither too thick nor too rare, but being
temper'd with both, fhine with a perpetual
Light, yet not equally glittering. *Albertus,*
however, makes the Saphirine Jacinth to
hold the firft Place; this is yellow and lucid,
has very little Aquofity in it, and is the
Ethiopic. Some fancy that the Granate,
which abide the Fire, and fhine with a
Violet Colour, are better. The Citron have
but little Red. The worft Sort of all are the
blue and azure, which have a fmall Red with
a thin Citron, yet they exceed the others
in Hardnefs, and are fcarce touch'd with the
Diamond; and thefe are the coldeft of all.
But other Species have Warmth and Drynefs
in the firft Degree. All are equal in Virtue,
tho'

tho' they differ in Colour. They invigorate animal Life, especially the Heart. They disperse Sorrow and imaginary Suspicions. They increase Ingenuity, Glory and Riches; are a Defence against Lightning and Enemies; and a Security to Travellers, so that no Pestilence in any Country shall hurt them, it raises Men to noble Honours, and preserves from Epidemical Distempers. *Aristotle*, indeed, holds, that they prepare Women for a Miscarriage.

Jasper, *Iaspis* as it is in the *Greek*, and in the *Latin*, Green, because the Green are the best, and valued above others, is a Stone of a green Colour, as we said, with a kind of Thickness, having red Veins, of which there are many Species. Some are translucent in a thick Green, and there are some green, marked with bloody Spots; others are red like a Tile, some are not much unlike red Porphyry. They are varied into so many Colours, that seventeen Species have been discover'd by the Learned, and by some more. For in these Times *Germany* is so fruitful of Jaspers, and produces such a Variety, that it would be in vain to reckon them; for our Design is to speak only of the nobler Sort And as we before intimated that the green Emeralds with red Veins were

more

more valuable than the reſt, eſpecially when they have a kind of Tranſparency; after theſe, the green, clear, ſtained with red, the dark red follow thoſe. The Citron are the worſt of all, but all are of equal Virtue. Being carry'd about one, it drives away the Fever and Dropſy, clears the Sight, expels noxious Phantaſms, reſtrains Luxury, and prevents Conception But eſpecially the green with Saffron Veins, which helps Women that are pregnant or in Labour It makes the Bearer of it victorious, powerful, and agreeable. But in all its Species, its principal Virtue is to ſtop the Flux of Blood whenceſoever it ariſes, it ought to be ſet in Gold, becauſe that increaſes its Virtues

Iris, is a Stone of a cryſtalline Colour, found in the Red Sea on the Coaſt of *Arabia*, and now in the Mountains of *Germany* in the River *Phenus*, it is of a Sexagonal Form, and is exceeding hard. If one Part of it is held in the Rays of the Sun, and the other Part in the Shade, under a Roof, it throws Beams, like thoſe of the Rainbow, on the oppoſite Wall, and from thence took its Name.

Ideus, is a Stone of an Iron Colour, it is found in *Ida*, a Mountain of *Crete*, from whence it derived its Name, it is in Shape like a Man's Thumb.

Ifciftos, or *Ifcultos*, is a Stone of a Saffron Colour, and found in a Part of *Spain*, near the *Gades* of *Hercules*, or, as now called, the Ifland of *Cales*. Some fay it is the fame as the *Amantes*, as it has the fame Virtue.

Indica, is of a ruddy Colour, and in the bruifing is purple. Another of the fame Name is of a white Afpect. It took its Name from the Place where it was found, its Virtue is not mention'd

Judaicus, fo called from *Judæa*, and is the fame as the *Cogolitus*.

Jovis, is a Gem, white, tender, and not ponderous

Ion, is of a Violet Colour, and is found in *India*

Jaguntia, which fome will have to be the *Granate*.

Ierarchites, is the fame as *Hierarchites*.

K

Kabrates, or *Kekabres*, is in Colour like Cryftal, with a dufky Whitenefs, whofe Virtue is, to render a Man eloquent and chearful, it gives Honours, Benevolence,

and

and defends him from Evil Cafualties It likewife cures the Dropfy.

Kamam, or *Kakaman*, is a white Stone diftinguifhed with various Colours, and is fo called from *Kaumate*, becaufe it carries Fire. It is found in fulphurous and hot Places, and very frequently mixed with the *Onyx* It has no determinate Virtue, but takes its Virtue from the Sculptures and Images that are en-grav'd upon it.

Karabe, is the fame as the *Succinum*, of which hereafter. Some however make a Difference between them, yet neither in Colour nor Virtue do they differ, but the Perfume of it moves the Epilepfy.

Kenne, it is faid, is bred in the Eyes of Stags in the Eaftern Parts; its Virtue is good againft Poifons.

Kimedini Limphatici, is the fame as the *Cimedia*.

Kinocetus, is a Stone not wholly ufelefs, fince it will caft out Devils

L

Lichinus, or *Lychinites*, is reckon'd among the burning Gems, it is red, and generated in many Places, the beft is among the *Indians*. It is called *Lichinus*, becaufe it er cites the Force of Light, and being kindled is itself a Candle. There are said to be two Species of it The first, as we said, and by some is affirmed, is a kind of flack Carbuncle. But the other borders upon a purple Colour, which being heated by the Sun, or by Friction, attracts Straws. It is hard and with Difficulty engraved; and when its Sculpture is impress'd on Wax, it holds it fast, as if a Beast had snatch'd it up with a Bite. Some say there are four Species of it; but the specifical ones I do not find

Lyncurius, is a Stone generated out of the Urine of the *Lynx,* and is harden'd by Time. It is found where those Animals frequent, and especially in some Parts of *Germany.* They say there are three Species of it, one whereof is sparkling like the Carbuncle. Another is Saffron inclining to a Darkness. The third is green The Virtue of it is, to assuage the Pain in the Stomach, to cure the Jaundice, to stop a Flux, and is good for the King's Evil

Lyncis, is also a Stone generated of the Urine of the Animal of its own Name, but differs from those above mention'd, when it is in the Earth it is soft, but when put in a cry Place, it hardens. Its Colour is white mixed with black closing with one another

While

While it is kept in the Earth or in a moist
Place before it is made dry, it generates
Mushrooms. The Virtue of this Stone, or
of the Mushrooms, is to help such as are
troubled with the Gravel or Stone; it takes
away the Pain of the Stomach, allays the
Flux of the Belly, and cures Fits of the
Mother

Lippares, or *Liparia*, is a Stone to which
all Kinds of Animals come of their own
Accord, as it were by a natural Instinct.
Some say, that he who has this Stone, needs
no other Invention to catch wild Beasts; it
is frequently found in *Iybia*. Others say,
that it has a wonderful Virtue in defending
Animals. For when a Beast is pursued by
Dogs and the Hunters, he hastens to find out
this Stone, to which he flies as to his Pio-
tector and Defender. For so long as the
Animal looks upon the said Stone, neither
the Dogs nor the Huntsman can see, which
if it be so, is indeed very strange; yet it is
affirmed by the Learned, and as to this, I
believe the Saying of *Pliny* is very true,
That there is no Lie so impudent which is
not vouch'd by Authority.

Limacie, is a Stone which took its Name
from the Animal in whose Head it is found.
It is extracted from the Head of a Snail

without

without a Shell, whofe Abode is in damp
and rocky Places. It ought to be drawn
out the Inftant it is feen, by fqueazing the
Head. It is of a white Colour, and but
little tranfparent, fmall, and like a Piece of
a Man's Nail. They fay, if it be hung
about the Neck, it cures one of a Fever.

Lacteus, is a Stone known by its citron
Colour; if bruifed in a Mortar with any
Liquor, it turns to a milky white. If
applied to rheumatic Eyes, it ftops the Courfe
of the Humours; it likewife avails in the
Beginning of Impoftumes of hot Eyes.

Leucoptalmus, is of four Colours, and has
the Likenefs of a Wolf's Eye, from whence
it took its Name. Some think it is the
fame as the *Obtallius*.

Lifimacus, is a Stone of the Marble Kind,
having Veins like golden Drops.

Leucocrifos, is a Stone of a green Colour
girded about with white Veins. Some take
it to be a Species of the *Emerald*, and is
reckoned under that Head.

Limoniates, is a green Stone in the Similitude of an *Emerald*, but not of fo much
Greennefs and Tranfparency.

Ligurius, as fome fancy, is like the *Elec-
torius*, and draws Straws. It appeafes the
Pain of the Stomach, ftops the Flux of the
Belly,

Belly, cures the Jaundice, sharpens the Sight, and by Physicians is rank'd among the Remedies for the Eyes.

Lignites, is a beautiful Stone, of the Colour of Glass, being hung about a Child, it preserves it from Witchcraft, and from the hellish Practices of a certain Sort of Women commonly called Witches. Being bound about the Forehead, it stops a Bleeding at the Nose, restores the Loss of the Senses, and helps to foretel future Events.

Lepidotes, is a Stone like the Scale of a Fish, and has divers Colours.

Limphicus, is a Stone of great Virtue. If wrapp'd in Silk, it is a Preservative against all Distempers in the Eyes, Jaws, Throat, a Cough and Head-ach, not only at present, but for the future.

Logdinus, is a Stone of a curious Whiteness, not exceeding the Bigness of a Bason or Bowl; it was first found in *Arabia*. But *Asia* affords a Coralline Sort, of a Size not larger than two Cubits; there is also found in the same Country a white Sort somewhat like Ivory.

Lauraces, are the Stones which cure the Head-ach.

Lychnitem, is a Kind of shining Marble, very white.

Laxo-

Lazolus, is a Stone placed under the Head of *Zumemelazoli*

Litos, is the fame as the Magnet.

Leucoftyctos, is the fame as Porphiry.

Lunarius, the fame as the *Selenites.*

M.

Margarita, or Pearl, has the firft Place among white Gems, generated by celeftial Dew in fome Sea Shell Fifh, as is held by Authors. Thefe Shell-Fifh, it's reported, early in a Morning, at a certain Seafon of the Year, leave the Bottom of the Sea, to draw in the Air, of which Pearls are generated ; and according to the Clearnefs of the Air taken in, Pearls are either lucid or muddy. The Pearl is for the moft part round, and by fome is called an *Onion* ; but there is only one of them found in one Shell And if by the Abundance of the Air taken in, there are more than one generated in a Shell, they are all globous, of which I have feen feven together, yet all in an oppofite Light fhew'd their Roundnefs , three or four are often feen, the moft perfect of which are thofe of a Silver Colour with a kind of Clearnefs : As to its Bignefs, the Learned fay it never exceeds an Ounce. There are two

Species

Species of Pearls; one is oriental, whofe Colour is white like polifh'd Silver, with a Tranfparency on its Superficies; and this is the moft perfect. The other Species is called occidental, which are tranfported from the *Britifh* Sea, whofe Colour is dull with a certain Whitenefs, bordering on a golden. The Orientals are more perfect than all others, and when they are large and round are bored thro' by Art, fometimes they are naturally fo, but not regularly, and thefe arc vile and ufelefs as to Ornament, and differ from thofe that are not perforated; and this is what is faid about them: The perforated Pearls are more perfect and have lefs Stipticity than thofe that are not perforated. It would be ridiculous to affirm, that the Opinions of the moft Learned Doctors are without Meaning, when they fay in their Recipe's, Pearls perforated and not perforated, and that inftead of perforated, they fhould write, perforated by Art; whereas the Difference is wholly owing to Accident and not to Complexion. Therefore that we may not be led into an Error, and may judge better than the Unfkilful, we fhould know, That the Pearls which are perforated, are thofe which have lain a long while in the Shells, and being quite ripe are

fpew'd

spew'd out into the Sea, where by a long
Stay and a perfect Ripeness, they are perforated, and lofe their ftyptick Quality ; and
of thefe the Doctors muft be underftood,
when they fpeak of the perforated , and it
is certain, that thofe that are perforated, as
they are not ufeful for Ornament, are not
tranfpoited to us. But they who rightly underftand how to make the Trial, bring
the Pearls to the Galls, becaufe thofe which
are not perforated are more ftyptick than the
perforated. Pearls have alfo phyfical Virtues
exceeding the Commodioufnefs of Ornament ;
being boil'd in Meat they cure the Quartan
Ague , bruifed and taken with Milk they
heal putrid Ulcers ; and being fo taken wonderfully cleai the Voice. They comfort the
Heait, and give Relief in Pains of the
Stomach, and remove the Epilepfy , they
ftop the Flux of the Belly , if taken with
Sugar, they yield Help in peftilential
Fevers ; and render him who carries them
chafte.

Medus, took its Name from the Country
where it was firft found. This Stone is of
two Species, the black and the green ; but
the green is called *Medinus*. If the black is
put into a green Mortar, and diffolved with
the Milk of a Woman who has a Male
Child,

Child, and applied to the Eyes, it reſtores loſt Sight; but if diſſolved in the Milk of an Ewe, which has once had a Lamb, it cures the Gout, if bound on to the Places affected. Being taken thro' the Mouth, it is a pernicious Poiſon. But this Stone is deſervedly called the Giver of Death and Health The green, which is called *Medinus*, if bruiſed and mixed with Gall, a little of the Magnet and Rain-water, and put to the Eyes for ſeven Days, it nouriſhes the Sight, and makes them ſee Things the moſt minute and almoſt inviſible.

Marble, is a Stone well known, of which there are divers Species that take their Names from the Countries or Places where they are found. But the true Marble, moſt eſteem'd by the Antients, is the green, and from thence it took its Name, for Marble, both in *Greek* and *Latin*, ſignifies green But all the Species are not generated in wet Places, for ſome are cut out of the Mountains. Some are generated here and there in the Earth; ſuch as we have already frequently taken Notice of, and ſhall again have Occaſion to mention. At preſent we ſhall only repeat the Names of its Species with their Colours, their Virtues you will find under their proper Heads. The *Lacedemonian*

is

is green, and the moſt precious of all. The *Auguſtean* ſucceeds to this, and is found in *Egypt* having black Spots gathered round in a Knot. The *Ophitean*, which is black and white with Serpentine Spots. The *Purpurite* or Porphiry, which comes from *Egypt*, having a red Colour, with white ſhining Dots or globous Lines. The *Baſamite*, of an iron Colour, is found in *Ethiopia* and *Egypt* The *Thebaic* is white interſected with golden Veins or Drops. The *Syenite* is found at the City *Syene* The *Parian* is the whiteſt of all, and is bred in an Iſland of its own Name. The *Onithean* is found in the Mountains of *Arabia*, and no where elſe as ſome think. But in *Germany* there is the greateſt Quantity, which has the Colour of Alabaſter with ſmall white Veins. There are alſo the *Leſbian*, *Corinthian*, *Cariſtean*, *Numidian*, *Lucullean* which is found in *Chios*, the *Limenſian*, the black Ivory ſo called from the Elephant. The *Cararian*, ſo called from the Place, is white maculated with red and ſometimes black Spots. It is likewiſe found in many Places with divers and various Names; which it would be uſeleſs to relate, ſince in Colour and Beauty it is like thoſe above-mention'd.

Muri-

Murina, is a Stone of divers Colours joined together, as of the Purple, white and fiery, with a kind of Reflection of one on the other, such as we see in the celestial Bow ; it is found among the *Parthians* Some think it is generated of the Moisture of the Earth condensed by the Heat of the Sun Its Virtue is not assigned by the Learned , but is useful for making Vessels. For *Pompey* first brought Murine Vessels into *Italy,* which for their Beauty were highly valued.

Mirites, for Colour and Smell, is like Myrrh , being rubbed on Cloth, it emits the Odour of Spikenard with its Sweetness

Malachites, rises almost to the Lustre of an Emerald, with a thick Vigour without Transparency, and takes its Name from Mallows, as it has as it were the Colour of it. It is a soft Stone, and is found in *Arabia,* *Cyprus* and *Persia,* but differently , for the *Arabian* has the Colour of Mallows , the *Cyprian* is inclined to a Greyness , the *Persian* retains a Brass Colour with a certain Greenness. The Virtue of this Stone is to defend Infants from adverse Casualties, and preserve the Cradle from hurtful Fancies, that so Infants may grow up in all Prosperity.

Memphitis, so called from a City of its own Name in which it was first found,

some

some think this Stone is useful to Chyrurgeons; as its Virtue is more stupifying than Opium. For being taken in Drink, or bruised in Vinegar, and applied to the Members which are to be cut off or burnt, it makes them so insensible, that they feel scarce any Pain.

Magnes, or the *Loadstone*, has a surprizing and incredible Virtue , and unless we had been taught by Experience, what we are about to say upon it would be thought vain. It is a Stone of an Iron Colour somewhat blue, sometimes of a brown or a different Colour. It was first found among the *Troglodites*, on the Sea-Shore. Five Kinds of Magnets are reckon'd up by the Learned, which are of divers Colours and Virtues, *viz.* the *Ethiopic, Macedonian, Antiochian, Alexandrian,* and *Asiatic*; but the Antients set the highest Value on the *Ethiopic* Magnet. It took its Name from the Inventor of it ; in these Times it is found in many and divers Places. They say, that Navigation is dangerous to those Ships in which Iron is wrought, in the Places where the Magnet is generated, where, by Reason of the Iron, they are detained , which in my Opinion is a ridiculous Notion. The Virtue of it, as I said, is stupendous and admirable, and if we

were

were not convinced by the Ufe of it, thofe
Things which are related about it we fhould
think were incredible. In attracting Iron, it
feems to have a kind of animal Virtue, and
that not only in Attraction, but in imprinting
its Virtue on it with a fort of Symboleity.
For Iron, touch'd by the *Magnet*, draws to
itfelf another Iron Body, as if it were another *Magnet*. It feems to contend with the
Diamond, for when the *Diamond* is put to it,
it does not attract Iron. Garlick likewife
binds up its Virtue. We can give no Reafon
for this, fince Philofophers are ignorant of
it, who only fay, that it proceeds from an
occult Property. I find there are three
Species, one which attracts Iron only, another which draws to itfelf human Flefh; and
a third, which is called *Hymmo*, which on
one Side draws Iron, and on the other drives
it away; and this only is with us, the reft
we have not feen It throws Iron from it in
this Manner; for Iron that is touch'd by one
Part of the *Magnet* is drawn to it, and the
oppofite Part being offered, is driven away,
as Experience fhews by a Needle hung to a
Thread. Navigation thro' the high Seas
would be dangerous were it not for the Virtue
and Knowledge of this Stone. It is an Index
to Navigators in their failing, as often as the

Star,

Star, which is their Guide, is hid with obscuring Clouds, without it they would be at a perfect Lofs in failing. The firft Navigators, who were wholly ignorant of the Art of the Compafs, fitted a Needle to a Straw or Bit of Wood crofs wife, and put it in a Bafon with Water, that the Needle might fwim; then they drew a *Magnet* round the Bafon, the Needle conftantly followed it; but the *Magnet* being taken away, the Point of the Needle, as if by a kind of natural Motion, turned in a Direction to the Star of the Arctic Pole Having thus learnt the Place of the Star, they directed their Motion accordingly. The Moderns, as they are ingenious, and as it is eafy to improve an Invention, framed the Compafs; in which they not only difcern the Place of the Arctic Pole, but all Parts of the Heaven, and the Winds. In the *Magnet* this is wonderful, that it has in it the Virtue of all the Parts of the Heavens, and according to the correfpondent Part of Heaven, thus by touching the Iron, it makes the Needle in the Mariner's Compafs, be turned to that Part of Heaven; and this is held by *Albertus Magnus* in his Book of the *Magnet*, and what I have often feen verified by Practice. Some call it the Sacred Stone;

and

and befides thefe wonderful Things which
we have related of it, there are more
Virtues which the Great Creator has given
to it. For being carried about one, it
cures the Cramp and Gout In the Hour of
Travail, if held in the Hand, it facilitates the
Birth. If bruifed and taken with Honey, by
purging, it cures the Dropfy And being
applied in the fame Manner, it affords
Relief to Wounds from poifon'd Iron. Being
taken with the Juice of Fennel, it helps the
Splenetick , and the Head being anointed
with it, it cures Baldnefs The Quantity of
a Dram, with the Fat of a Serpent, and the
Juice of Nettles, if given to any one to carry,
makes him mad, and drives him from his
Kindred, Habitation and Country. This
Stone alfo difcovers adulterous Wives ;
for if it be fecretly hid in the Bed under the
Head of the fleeping Wife, if fhe is chafte,
the Hufband embraces her, but if adulterous,
fhe immediately jumps out of the Bed fleeping as if forced by a horrible Stink. But
being carried about one, it reconciles Wives
to their Hufbands, and Hufbands to their
Wives. It takes away Fears and Jealoufies.
It makes a Man gracious, perfuafive, and
elegant in his Converfation Again ; if it
be bruifed to Powder, and ftrewed over

Coals in the Corners of the House, as the Smoak flies upward, they who are in the House prefently run away, imagining that the whole House is falling; and fo terrified are they with Fancies, that they fly out, leaving every Thing behind them; and by this Artifice Thieves feize on Goods by the commodious Flight of the Owners. It is reported by fome, that by this Stone the Walls and Shell of a certain Temple, the Floor being taken away, were upheld; within which an Idol made of Iron, of a thoufand Pounds Weight, was hung fufpended in the Air by Virtue of the Loadftone. The Sum of the Matter is this, that if the Heads and Points of many Needles were rubbed on this Stone, only by the Joining of one to the other, they might be all held up by the firft fufpended in the Air.

Magnafia, or *Magnofia,* is of a black Colour, and ufeful in the Art of Glafs-making. It is the fame as the *Alabandicus.*

Marchafites, of which there are many and divers Species; and they are varied according to the Diverfity of Metals. For fome are Gold, fome Silver, others Copper, and others Iron; and they are diverfified in the Colour according to the Species of the Metal

of

of which it is. This the Alchymifts know very well. It is not liquified by Fire, but is burnt by itfelf. Some call it the Stone of Light, becaufe it gives Relief in loft Sight. Some fay, it is called the Stone of Light, becaufe when ftruck with a Steel it makes Fire, and in apt Matter kindles it.

Medea, is a Stone which took its Name from the Invention of the Witch *Medea.* It has a black Colour with golden Veins, and if bruifed in Water, yields the Tafte of Wine with a Saffron Colour.

Morion, is a *Cyprian* and *French* Stone, exceeding black and very tranfparent, fit for Grave-Stones.

Mitridax, is a *Perfian* Stone, which being play'd on by the Sun, fhines with various Colours.

Melites, or *Melitites,* which when pounded in Water, yields a fweet Tafte, and gives Help in various Diforders, as is held by many learned Men, particulaily *Pliny.*

N

Nitre, is numbred by the Learned among Stones, altho' it is not one, as we faid of many others. It is of the Colour of Salt and clear. It has the Virtue both of dif-

folving

folving and attracting. It is made out of the Saltnefs of the Earth where Beafts and Men have promifcuoufly mingled. It's notorious how great its Virtue is in warlike Inftruments in throwing Stones; for when it is kindled by Fire, it rarifies, and is violently dilated , by which Means it drives out the Stones and whatever ftops its Vent. It was never found out by the Antients; modern Induftry invented it. Of three Things proportionally mixed, a certain Compofition is made, which no Force can withftand; for it breaks, leads, drives, and deftroys all Things.

Nicolus, is of a double Colour , its Superficies is yellow, and its Infide black. Some think it is a Species of the *Calcedonius*. They fay, it took its Name from a *Greek*. Its Virtue is to render the Bearer of it victorious and grateful to the People.

Naffonites, is a Stone of a fanguin Colour, marked or fhaded with black Veins , it is found in Quickfands

Nemeffitis, is an excellent Stone, which they fay the *Athenians* took from the Altar of the Goddefs *Nemefia*.

Nofe, or *Nifus*, is the fame as *Alabaftrides*.

Onix,

O

Onyx, is a Stone which has the Colour of a human Nail; for fo it fignifies both in *Greek* and *Latin*. It is tranfparent, and feldom found alone Its Species is varied from the Diverfity of Colours with which it is joined, and from the Place where it is found Some fay there are two Species of it; others, that there are five. The firft, which is the true, is that which we have already mentioned Another Sort they fay is of an exceeding black Colour. The third is black with white Veins or Circles, and this *Arabia* fends us. *India* produces an *Onyx* that is reddifh with white Veins. The fifth has a Mixture of the black and reddifh Colour. Some fay, that the true *Onyx* has the Colour of the *Amethyft*, the *Carbuncle*, and the *Crifolete*, which Colours are mixed with White and Black. This Stone reprefents many horrible Things in Sleep. He who carries it about him, ftirs up Quarrels and Contentions. It increafes Spittle in Children, and haftens a Birth. Being hung about the Neck of one who has the Epilepfy, it prevents his falling. This wonderful Property s faid to be in the *Onyx*; that, being ap-

plied

plied to a weak Eye, it enters it of its own Accord, as if it were a fenfible Thing, and goes round it without any Trouble, and if it finds any Thing within that is noxious, it drives it out and tempers the hurtful and contrary Humours.

Onicinus, tho' it is a Gum from a Tree of its own Name, is yet number'd among Stones, and is harden'd in the fame Manner as Amber is faid to be. Its Colour is white mixed with a moderate red If put upon a live Coal, in the Manner of Incenfe, it gives a fweet and fragrant Smell, it whitens the Hards, and cures the Itch.

Opalus, Opal, is a Stone wonderful to behold, as it is compos'd of many and divers Colours of fhining Gems, as of the *Carbuncle, Amethift, Emerald,* and many others, with a Variety equally glittering and admirable to fee. It is found only in *India* ; and is not bigger than a large Filbert. How highly it was valued by the Antients, we are informed by *Pliny,* in his 37th Book, who fays, it was eftimated at 20,000 Sefterces, which amounts to fomething more than 200£ Sterling. Its Virtue prevails againft all the Difeafes of the Eyes. It fharpens and ftrengthens the Sight. It cannot be improper to attribute to it fo

many

many Virtues, since it partakes of the Nature and Colour of so many Stones

Obtalius, or *Obtalmius*, whose Colour is not affign'd by the Learned, altho' some fay it is of many Colours. Wonderful is its Virtue in preferving the Eyes from various Diftempers. It fharpens the Sight of him that carries it, but darkens thofe of the Byftanders, fo that they are not able to fee. If it be wrapt in a Leaf of Laurel, and a Charm faid over it, and carried cautioufly, it has a wonderful Effect.

Orites, is a Stone which we fay has three Species, one black of a round Figure. This being bruifed and mixed with Oil of Rofes, perfectly cures the Wounds, given by wild Beafts, and poifonous Bites, and keeps him who carries it unhurt among all Sorts of wild Beafts. There is another *Orites* which is green, fprinkled with white Spots; this preferves him who carries it from adverfe Cafualties. The third Species is thin like a Plate of Iron, ftrewed with a few Drops. Being hung about the Neck, it fuffers not Women to conceive; but if they are pregnant makes them mifcarry

Orphanus, is of a violet Colour. It is of fuch Beauty and Value, that the *Roman* Emperors fet it in their Crowns. It fhines

in

in the Dark. It is called *Orphan*, becaufe at that Time, there was only one of them found. It is highly efteemed by Emperors, becaufe it preferves their regal Honours.

Obfius, or *Obfianus*, is of a black tranfparent Colour in the Likenefs of Glafs, when it is made even and polifh'd, it reflects Shades and Images like a Looking-glafs, and for its Beauty is put in the Walls of Edifices. It is found in *Lybia*, *Germany*, and *India*

Oftracites, is a Stone of the Likenefs of an Oyfter-fhell, from which it took its Name; it is ufed as the Pumice to fmooth the Skin. Its Virtue is, if given in Drink, to ftop Bleeding If pounded with Honey, it affwages Pains in the Breafts.

Ophites, is as before obferv'd, of the Marble Kind, and has ferpentine Spots, from which it had its Name There are two Species of it, the foft, which is white, and the brown which is hard and greenifh, and fprinkled with Saffron Spots. The Antients embellifh'd the Walls of their Houfes with it. Its Virtue is, if hung about the Neck, to allay the Pains of the Head, and gives Relief to thofe who are ftung with Serpents. The White, we think, reftores Health to the Lunatic and Lethargic. It is had in *Germany*,

and

and they make drinking Veffels of it. Some
hold that the *Ophites* was the Stone of which
they made Cauldrons. By Reafon of its
Softnefs, it is turned and cut, and in the
Province of *Holland*, they faw it into Plates
for the Covering of Houfes , but it hardens
by Fire.

Oftratias, is a Stone like a Jacynth, but
harder , and its Hardnefs is liken'd to the
Adamant.

Ophicardelon, in *Greek* fignifying the Heart
of a Serpent, is a black Stone divided with
two white Lines

Okitokius, is a Stone lefs than the *Ethices*,
and, like that, refounds from within , it has
a fmooth Surface, and is foon broken Phyficians diffolve it in the Juice of certain
Herbs, and make an Ointment of it which
has this peculiar Property, that by dipping
the Finger in it, and touching any Wood,
Metal, or Stone, tho' ever fo hard, it will
inftantly break it.

Onagari, is the fame as the *Afinius*, of
which we have fpoke before *Onager* both
in *Greek* and *Latin*, fignifies a wild Afs.

Ombria, is the fame as *Ceraunia*, of which
before.

Ornicus, is the fame as the *Sapphire*.

Olea,

Olea, is a Stone of a yellow, green, and white Colour.

P

Prassius, is so called from an Herb of its own Name, as being somewhat like it in Colour. They say that the *Prassius* is the House of the *Emerald* It's said to be generated in *Ethiopia* in the River *Nile*. There are three Species of it. One, as I said, is of a dull Green, transparent, but not clear. Another is green, impress'd with sanguin Drops. The third is green, lined with white Junctures or *Calcedonian* Marks ; it is of no small Virtue , it comforts the Sight , and has all the Virtues of the *Emerald* tho' diminutively.

Panthera, is a Stone which is also called *Evantus* It has various Colours mixed in one Body in Similitude of the Animal of its own Name, which it takes from the Variety of its Colours. Such a *Stone* has in it certain black, red, pale, green, rosy and purple Marks It is found in the Country of *Media*. If you look on it by the rising Sun, you will be succesful in all your Actions of that Day. They say it has as many Virtues as it

has

has Mixtures of other Stones; for every Stone gives it its own Virtue.

Pontica, is a Gem tranfparent with a Bluenefs. I find three Species of it particularly noted. It takes its Name from *Pontus*, where it is found, and alfo from the Likenefs of its Water. With its Bluenefs it has red Stars, or is fprinkled over with fanguin Drops. Another Sort fhines with golden Marks; and a third is ftreaked with long red Lines mixed with blue. It's faid, that by it the Devil is interrogated and put to Flight, and is compell'd to return Anfwers to him that afks any Queftions.

Peantes, or *Peantides*, is a Stone which fome fay, has the Female Sex; that at a certain Time it conceives, and brings forth one like itfelf. But tho' this is written by fome, it does not pleafe me, I rather think that fuch Writers have fell into an Error by mifunderftanding the Words of the Antients. For when they fay fuch a Stone is of the Female Sex, they don't mean that that Stone can conceive, but that it affords Help to Women in their Conception and bringing forth. Which of thefe Opinions is the trueft, I fubmit to the Judgment of the Learned. The Colour of this Stone is like Water congealed with Cold.

Py

Pyrites, fo called from *Pyr*, which fignifies Fire, and is vulgarly termed the Fire-ftone; for when it is ftruck with a Steel, it flafhes Fire. But by fome it is called *Ypeftionus*, that is, *Vulcan* Hence, in a large Senfe, all Stones that ftrike Fire may be called *Pyrites*. The *Marchafite*, from its producing Fire, is likewife called *Pyrites* The *Coral* alfo, from its deep Rednefs, by fome is called *Pyrites*. The true *Pyrites* is that which with a quick Stroke produces Fire, is of a yellow Colour, very blunt and thick, by the wafhing of the Sea it is finely polifh'd, and as it were regulaily rude. But *Diofcorides* affirms it is of the Colour of Brafs, which being bruifed and held hard between the Fingers of the Right Hand, burns it It is found in many Places It is faid to be of great Ufe in Medicine, and particularly for Diftempers of the Eyes as the Learned hold

Phrigius, took its Name from the Province of its own Name in which it was firft found. It is likewife found in *Cyprus* The Colour of it is pale, and it is moderately heavy, like Punic Earth Being thrice heated and befprinkled with Wine, it grows red, and is of ufe in colouring Cloth. We have found it in a threefold Species. One is that already mention'd. Another is like

burnt

burnt Brafs, and is the Drofs of Brafs. There is a third tho' it be not a true one, becaufe it is artificial, and made of the *Pyrites* by Calcination in the Furnace, till it acquires a fanguin Colour, yet it is reckon'd in the Species of the *Phrigius*. Its Virtue is Stiptic, and reduces proud Flefh in Wounds. It cures feeding and malignant Ulcers, and affuages the Flux of the Eyes.

Porphyry, is a blunt Stone, ponderous, very hard, of a reddifh Colour, marked with fmall white Spots, of which we have fpoke above under the Head of *Marble*, as it is of that Species It was much in Ufe among the Antients in the building of Edifices.

Podros, is one of the burning Gems, and for its Whitenefs obtains the firft Place after the Pearl

Panconus, is of a cryftal Colour, not exceeding the Bignefs of a Finger, and is of an oblong Figure ; but differs from the Cryftal, becaufe it wants Angles.

Punicus ; there are two Species of this Stone, which is found in the *Æolian* Ifles ; that which is white and heavy is the moft perfect Its Efficacy is powerful in Medicines. For being burnt, wafhed and dried, it is very good for the Eyes It cleanfes Wounds and fkins over Sores. It prevents Drunkennefs.

nefs, if taken before drinking Wine.

Præconiſſus, is of a Colour as it were almoſt wholly Saphiiine; it is however blunt and cloſe with *Calcedonian* Marks, and delights the Eyes with its agreeable Embelliſhments.

Pavonius, is a Stone, which being given in Drink with a moderate Sweat, forces the Perſon who takes it into all the Fire of Love.

Pumex, or the Pumice Stone, is known to every Body, porous, and exceeding light and tender. It is, however, very often a chemical, and ſometimes a phyſical Stone; and not unuſeful to Writers.

Paragonius, is double, black and golden; the black is uſed in attaining the Knowledge of Metals, as Goldſmiths know, when they bring the Metals to it.

Pheonicites, is a Stone in the Likeneſs and Colour of an Acorn.

Philoginos, is the ſame as the *Criſites.*

Q

Quirinus, or *Quirus,* is a juggling Stone, found in the Neſt of the Hoopoop. The Virtue of it is, that if it is laid on the Breaſt of one who is ſleeping, it forces him to diſcover his Rogueries.

Quai-

Quaidros, is the fame as the *Vulturis*; of which hereafter.

R

Radaim, is a Stone black and tranfparent. It is found in the Head of a Cock, altho' fome fay, it is found in the Head of a Sea Cat, as we before obferv'd under the Head of *Doriatides*. When it is cut off fuddenly, and put in a Place to be eat by Pifmires, after the Flefh is confum'd, it is found. It gives Favour and Honours to him that wears it, and is a Help in governing.

Ranius, *Rabri*, *Rami*, all fynonimous, and according to fome, is the fame as *Bolus Armenus*, but feems to differ from it, for it is of a livid Colour, and borders upon white with a Clearnefs. It is weighty, and its Virtue is to refift Poifon, like the *Bolus Armenus*.

Rubinus, *Ruby*, is a Species of the Carbuncle as we have faid; nor differs from it but in Quantity, and has the like Virtue; of which there are two Species. One is that of which we have already fpoken, the other is darker, and but of fmall Value.

Sapphire,

S

Sapphire, is a Stone of a yellow or Skie-blue Colour, perfpicuous like the moft pure Azure, and the deeper Yellownefs it is with a Tranfparency, the more perfect. But that is the moft precious, which being play'd on by the Sun emits as it were a burning Brightnefs, and there is never the leaft Image perceived in it It is found about the *Lybian* Quickfands, but the *Indians* have better. Some call it the Jewel of Jewels for its Beauty, and on Account of its Colour; tho' others fay, it claims this Name, not for its Colour, but its Virtue. It refrefhes the Body, and gives a good Colour; it checks the Ardor of Luft, and makes a Perfon chafte and virtuous, and reftrains too much Sweat. It takes away the Filth of the Eyes and the Pains of the Head. Being drank with Milk, it appeafes the Gripes of the Belly. It renders the Bearer of it pacifick, amiable, pious and devout, and confirms the Soul in good Works. It difcovers Frauds; expels Terrors. It is of great Service in magic Arts, and is faid to be of prodigious Efficacy in the Works of Necromancy. It difcharges a Carbuncle with a fingle Touch.

The

The Eyes being touch'd with it, it preferves them from being injur'd by the Small-Pox.

Smaragdus, or Emerald, of which there are many Kinds ; but the Scythian obtains the firft Place of them all Its Greennefs is fo intenfely, that it is not only not dulled when put under any Light or the Beams of the Sun, but is fuperior to all Force, and ftains the encircling Air with its Greennefs ; and from hence it has its Name , for every deep Green may , be called an Emerald. I find twelve Species of it defcribed by Lapidaries But, as we faid, the Scythian are more precious and noble than the reft , the Britifh are the next, the Egyptian, Hermician, Perfian, and fome that are found in Copper-Mines But tho' all thefe are tranfparent, yet they differ in the Deepnefs of their Green. And fo delightful is their Colour, that there is fcarce any Jewel that affords a more grateful Refrefhment to the Eyes And when the Face of it is evened, it reflects Images like a Looking-glafs. It is reported that Nero Cæfar had an Emerald of a furprizing Bignefs, in which he beheld the Combats of the Gladiators. There are other Species of them of divers Colours, and variegated with little Spots, which are called Falfe Emeralds, which, with the fore-mention'd,

K   make

make up the Number Twelve. The six Species above-named are not, however, so remarkable for their Largeness, as are those of the *False Emerald,* an Obelisk of which *Pliny* gives an Account of, that was fifty Cubits high; of one that was four Cubits high; of another of two, in the Temple of *Jupiter,* in the Possession of the King of *Babylon. Theophrastus* says, he had seen an Emerald of four Cubits. It's reported that at *Rome* there was a large one in the Temple of *Hercules.* But, as before observed, there is no great Quantity of those that are perfect. But such is the Form of *Emeralds,* that their Faults cannot be discover'd in their Superficies, as the Colour is equally fulgent, and Images impressed. Many Virtues are fabled of it.

Succinum, or *Amber,* is a Species, as before observ'd of the *Gagates,* altho' it is a Gum. For its Beauty, and the Use of it by the Antients, it is number'd among Gems. It is yellow, transparent, and has in it a kind of Blueness mixed with a Cast of the Saffron. Of what Esteem it was among the Antients, we may learn from *Pliny.* It is said to be the Gum of a Tree of its own Name, not unlike a Pine-tree. It appears however that it is not *Gummi Populi,* as the Poets imagine from the Fable of *Phaeton.* It is found in

many

many Places, as in *Dacia, England, Bretagne,* But the greatest Plenty of it is in some Islands on the Shore of the Northern Ocean, on the Side of *Germany.* The Gum is condens'd in this Climate, by the Severity of Cold, and by Length of Time. But as it mostly oozes out of Trees, whatever extraneous Matter it finds, is inclosed in the Gum. Hence it is we often see buried in it small Animals, Straws, *&c* and sometimes Deceivers will soften the Amber and put into it some extraneous Matter. When this Gum is harden'd on the Trees, and they are shook by a Gust of Wind, if near the Sea, it falls into it ; and there is more harden'd, and becomes more shining; at length it is driven by Tempest on Shore, and is taken up by Nets. And as the *Magnet* attracts Iron, so Amber, when heated by being rubbed on Cloth, draws Straws The Virtues of Amber are the same as those of the *Gagates,* tho' more numerous and powerful. It naturally restrains the Flux of the Belly ; is an efficacious Remedy for all Disorders in the Throat, to prevent which the Antients made the Women and Children wear it in Bracelets and Necklaces. It is good against Poison. If laid on the left Breast of a Wife when she is asleep, it makes her confess all

K 2

her evil Deeds. Being taken inwardly, it provokes Urine, brings down the Menfes, and facilitates a Birth. It faftens Teeth that are loofen'd, and by the Smoak of it, poifonous Infects are driven away If we would difcover whether a Woman has been corrupted, let it be laid in Water for three Days, and then fhewn to her, and if fhe is guilty, it will immediately force her to make Water.

Sardius, or *Sarda*, is numbred among the burning Gems, yet the baleft Sort of them was moft in Ufe among the Antients. It is of a red or bloody Colour, but is darker and duller than the *Cornelian*. It has the fixth Place in the Diftinction of Colours It was firft found in *Sardinia*, from whence it took its Name. There are counted five Species of it, but the *Babylonian* exceeds them all The *Indian* is next, then the *Arabian*, *Egyptian*, and laftly the *Cyprian*. In many Places where they cut out Stones, it is found in the Middle of them as it were a Heart, as in the Ifland *Paros*. The Males fhine brighter than the Females, for the Females are the fatteft and glitter more obfcurely It bind's up the *Onyx*, for when it is prefent, the other cannot hurt. It caufes horrid Dreams in Sleep It increafes Wealth,

Wealth; gives Cheaifulnefs, whets the Wit; reftrains the Bloody Flux, and gives Conqueft over Enemies. Some think the *Sardius* is the *Cornelian*, which is a falfe Notion.

Sardonyx, or *Sardonius*, is a Stone compounded of the *Sardius* and *Onyx*, and very often alfo of the *Chalcedonius* Sometimes it is diftinguifhed with three Colours, black, *Calcedonian*, and *Sardian*, and the more diftinct the Colours are, fo much the better is the *Sardonyx* In former Times it was highly valued by the antient *Romans*. Its Virtue is to put a Reftraint on lafcivious Motions, and make a Man merry and agreeable. It is the beft of any for making Seals, as it does not ftick to the Wax

Selenites, *Sirites*, *Siderites*, are fynonimous Names of the fame Stone This Stone, fome fay, is tranfparent, with a clear and honeylike Brightnefs, and contains the Figure of the Moon or a clouded Star. It glitters in the Dark, and takes its Name from the Place where it was found. The Learned have allotted various Species to this Stone. The firft we have already given an Account of Another we have fpoke of under the Head of *Celonites*, as fome think it is of this Species. But the *Perfian* emulates the Greennefs of the *Jafper*, duely keeping the

Times

Times of the Lunar Motion, and as if anxious for some Damage sustain'd in the Heavens, its Colour increases or decreases with the Moon. It is very powerful in reconciling Love; and during the whole Time of the Increase of the Moon, it helps the Pthisical; but in the Decrease, it discovers surprising Effects, for it enables a Person to foretel future Events. Being put into the Mouth, which must be first washed with Water, such Affairs are thought of, as ought or ought not to be taken in Hand. If to be undertaken, they are so fixed on the Mind that they cannot be forgotten; but if not, they soon vanish out of the Mind.

Samius, is a Stone so called from the Island of its own Name; from its first Invention Artificers have used it to polish Gold. It is white, heavy and brittle. Its Virtue is to cure the Swimming of the Head and the Loss of the Understanding. But if it be taken in Drink, it prevents Abortion. If carried in the left Hand, it stops the Running of Tears of aged People, and gives Help in other Disorders of the Eyes, if bruised in Milk and applied to them.

Smirillus, is the File and Serpent of all Things, except the *Diamond*; it consumes and corrodes all Things. It is a Stone of an

iron

iron Colour and exceeding hard , it is found in many and divers Places. It is used for the cutting and plaining of Stones, and the scouring of Arms.

Syrius, is a Stone so called from *Syria.* While it is whole, it is not to be sunk in Water ; but being diminished, it goes to the Bottom. The Cause of this Effect is, that it holds Air included in it, and swims by the Lightness of the Air ; but when the Stone is broke, the Air is let out, and the Gravity of the Stone being only left, it sinks down.

Solis Gemma, the Jewel of the Sun, is of a bright white Colour, like the *Beril,* and when placed in the full Blaze of the Sun, it spreads about its shining Rays ; and from hence took its Name. It has a wonderful Efficacy against any deadly poisonous Draught.

Sagida, or *Sadida,* is a Stone of the Colour of the *Prassius* ; it has so great an Affection to cling about Vessels, that it will dart itself upward from the Bottom of the Sea, and stick so close to a Ship, that unless you cut away that Part of the Wood to which it adheres, it can scarcely be plucked off.

Sandastros, or *Sadasius,* is a Stone of an igneous Perspicuity, sprinkled as it were

K 4   with

with gold Drops, which feem like Stars, and the more Starry it is, or the greater Number of Drops it contains, which fhine from within, fo much the more precious it is accounted It is placed in the Number of burning Jewels. It took its Name from the Place where it was firft found *Arabia* like-wife produces it; it is fuppofed to be in Ufe in the Ceremonies of the *Chaldeans* It is faid to be Male and Female, and is diftinguifh-ed by the Colour A milder Flame is affigned to the Females, but a yellower and more fervent to the Males

Sarcofagus, is a Stone of which the Antients built their Monuments, and took its Name from its Effect. For *Sarcos*, in *Greek*, fignifies Flefh, *Fagos* to eat, from whence *Sarcofagis*, or devouring Bodies in a Coffin, for it confumes a human Body that is placed in it, infomuch that in forty Days the very Teeth are gone, fo that nothing appears Afterwards, not only all Monuments conftructed of that Stone, but all Sepulchers of Stone were called *Sarcofaga*. Nav, farther, if this Stone be bound to a Man while he is alive, it has the Force of eating away his Teeth.

Sefinus, is a Stone of an Afhy Colour, not

hard

hard It is ufeful in Cookery, of which they make Cauldrons Being daubed with Oil, it hardens in the Fire and turns black.

Siderites, is a Stone in Colour not much unlike Iron Its Virtue is, that if it be ufed in Sorceries, it excites Difcords.

Stuxites, is a Stone content with a moderate Beauty, but not fo in its Virtue, for if bruifed and flily given in Meat with Ragwort, it gives a prodigious Stiffnefs to the *Penis*, being hung about the Neck, it makes a good Digeftion, and infufes a Defire of Fruition

Samothracia, is a Stone of a black Colour and light, fomething like burnt Wood; it is fo called from the Ifland of its own Name. It is likewife found in our Mountains between *Fanum* and *Pijaro* under the Mountain *Catighan*, for under the Mountain is a black Vein, in which are contained thefe Stones, when they are put in Fire they give a Smell like Pitch, the Smoak of it avails in Fits of the Mother.

Spinella, is one of the burning Gems, as we obferved under the Head of *Carbuncle*; its Colour is more open and clear than the Colour of the *Ruby*, but in Virtue is like it, and by fome is called the *Rubith*

San-

Sanguineus Lapis, or the bloody-colour'd Stone, is the same as the *Ematites.*

Spongius, is a Stone the same as the *Cysteolithos.*

Senedeg, is the same as the *Ematrices.*

Sirites, the same as the *Sapphire.*

Specularis, is the same as the *Phengites.*

Sanctus Lapis, the holy Stone, the same as the *Sapphire.*

Sarda, the same as *Sardius.*

Simodontides, the same as *Corvina.*

T

Topatius, or *Topasion,* the *Topaz,* is a most splendid and famous Stone of those they call burning Gems, of which there are two Species; one of a yellow Colour bordering upon Gold, with some Greenness. This is oriental, defies the File, and is the best. The other is Western, greener than the other, has a slack Colour of the Gold, wastes by Use, suffers by the File, and is deemed the worst; and of this Species some think is the *Crysopteron.* This Stone was first found in an Island of *Arabia,* call'd *Chitis.* For some

Trog-

Troglodite Pyrates being driven there by a Tempeſt, and wanting Proviſion, they dug up Herbs and Roots for their Food, and found this Stone, and from this Accident it deriv'd its Name, for *Topaſion*, in the *Arabic* Tongue, is the ſame as Search. *Pliny*, however, is of a contrary Opinion as to the Impoſition of the Name. He relates that it was found in an Iſland of the Red Sea, at the Diſtance of about three Hundred Furlongs from the Shore, which lies naturally on a Deſcent and always beclouded with Fogs. It is ſought for by Mariners when they have no Light; and from this Searching it took the Name of *Topaz*. It's reported that *Ptolomy Philadelphus*, had a Topaz of three Cubits They ſay, that if the *Topaz* is thrown into Water boiling hot, it quickly cools, and that by this Coolneſs laſcivious Motions are quell'd. It's a Cure for the Phrenſy, cleanſes the Hemorrhoids, cures and prevents Lunacy, increaſes Riches, aſſuages Anger and Sorrow, and averts ſudden Death; Blood flowing from a Wound is ſtopped if this be bound over it, and it makes the Bearer of it obtain the Favour of Princes.

Turchion, or *Turcheſia*, the *Turcois*, is a yellow Stone bordering upon white, and if paſſed thro' Milk, is of a yellow Colour, is very agreeable to the Sight, and took its Name from the Country   There is a vulgar Opinion, that it is uſeful to Horſemen, and that ſo long as the Rider has it with him, his Hoſe will never tire him, and will preſerve him unhurt from any Accident. It ſtrengthens the Sight with its Aſpect. It is ſaid to defend him that carries it from outward and evil Caſualties

Trachius, is a Stone of which there are two Species, the black is ſonorous, and the other greeniſh, not tranſparent.

Thirſitis, is like the *Coral*   They ſay, if it be taken in a Draught, it brings on Sleep.

Talc Alchimicus, is a Stone, lucid, luminous, of the Colour of Silver, and by Sublimation becomes the worſt of Poiſons

Tartis, is a Stone of a very beautiful Colour, like a Peacock, noble, and moſt delightful to behold, nor is it leſs famous for its Virtue than its Aſpect

Tegolitus, is the ſame as *Cagolites*.

Trapendanus, is a Species of the *Pirites*.

Teſtos, the ſame as *Tegolitus*.

Varach,

V.

Varach, is a Stone not to be found among us It has the Virtue of ftopping every Kind of Flux , inftead of which Phyficians ufe *Dragon's Blood*

Vernix, or *Armenicus*, is a Stone, whofe Virtue is faid to afford Help to the Melancholy, the Splenetick, the Liver-grown, and thofe alfo who are troubled with the Cholick

Veientana Italica, has its Name from the Place It is alfo found in many other Places, and from thefe takes its Sir-name. It is a black Stone with white fhining Lines and Marks.

Vulturis, fo called from the Bird of its own Name, whofe Head being fuddenly cut off, it is found in the Brain. It gives Health to thofe who carry it. It fills a Woman's Breafts with Milk. It gives Succefs to thofe who petition for Favours.

Virites, is the fame as *Pyrites*.

Vetrachius, the fame as *Ranus*

Unio, the fame as the *Pearl*

Xiph.

X.

Xiphinos, is the fame as the *Sapphire*.

Y.

Yecticas, is a Stone of a fanguine Colour, hard and obfcure. It is of Ufe in trying Metals.

Ydrinus, and by fome called the *Serpentine*; it helps thofe who are troubled with Rheum, and frees the human Body from too much Humidity; it reftores dropfical Bodies to their priftine State, if they ftand three Hours with it in the Sun, for they will evacuate a moft foul Water by Sweat. They fay it muft be cautioufly us'd, for it will extract not only the extraneous Humidity, but alfo the natural and implanted Juices. It drives away poifonous Worms. If taken inwardly, it is faid to break the Stone in the Bladder.

Yfoberillus, is a Species of the *Beril*.

Zume-

Z.

Zumemellazuli, or *Zemech*, but in *Latin* is the Stone *Lazuli*. This Stone is yellow, of the Colour of the Sky when it is in its greateſt Serenity, not tranſparent, and ſhines with golden Streaks ; it ſuſtains the Fire, and from its Beauty is called the celeſtial or ſtarry Stone. Being prepared by Phyſicians, it cures melancholy Diſorders. There is alſo made of it a Colour call'd the Ultramarine Azure.

Zarites, has the Similitude of the Colour of Glaſs They ſay it ſtops Bleeding if hung about the Neck.

Ziazaa, took its Name from a Place ; it has a Mixture of white, black, and many other Colours, ſo that none of them remains perfectly diſtinguiſhable. It renders him who carries it litigious, and makes him ſee terrible Things in his Sleep.

Zmilaces, or *Zmilanthis*, is a Stone of a marble Colour, mixed with a Blue. It is found in the *Euphrates*, having in the Middle

dle of it a little Ball of a greyish Colour.

Zoronyfias, is said to be found in the River *Indus*; they say it was a Gem of the *Magi* And here we put an End to this Book.

F I N I S.

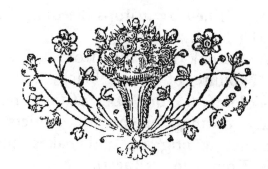

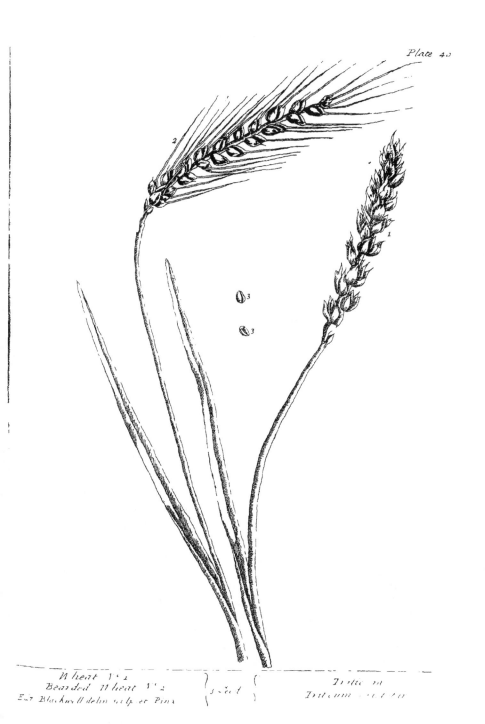

Plate 40

Wheat 1.1
Bearded Wheat 1.2
Eat Blackwell delin sculp et Pinx

Triticum
Triticum

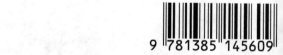